I0053426

Frontiers in Heart Failure

(Volume 3)

(Heart Failure in Pediatric Patients)

Edited by:
Mohammad El Tahlawi

Zagazig University Hospitals, Cardiology Department,
University St, Zagazig, Egypt

Frontiers in Heart Failure

Volume # 3

Editor: Mohammad El Tahlawi

ISSN (Online): 2468-8053

ISSN (Print): 2468-8045

ISBN (Online): 978-9-81141-090-1

ISBN (Print): 978-9-81141-089-5

© 2020, Bentham eBooks imprint.

Published by Bentham Science Publishers – Sharjah, UAE. All Rights Reserved.

BENTHAM SCIENCE PUBLISHERS LTD.
End User License Agreement (for non-institutional, personal use)

This is an agreement between you and Bentham Science Publishers Ltd. Please read this License Agreement carefully before using the book/echapter/ejournal (**"Work"**). Your use of the Work constitutes your agreement to the terms and conditions set forth in this License Agreement. If you do not agree to these terms and conditions then you should not use the Work.

Bentham Science Publishers agrees to grant you a non-exclusive, non-transferable limited license to use the Work subject to and in accordance with the following terms and conditions. This License Agreement is for non-library, personal use only. For a library / institutional / multi user license in respect of the Work, please contact: permission@benthamscience.net.

Usage Rules:

1. All rights reserved: The Work is the subject of copyright and Bentham Science Publishers either owns the Work (and the copyright in it) or is licensed to distribute the Work. You shall not copy, reproduce, modify, remove, delete, augment, add to, publish, transmit, sell, resell, create derivative works from, or in any way exploit the Work or make the Work available for others to do any of the same, in any form or by any means, in whole or in part, in each case without the prior written permission of Bentham Science Publishers, unless stated otherwise in this License Agreement.
2. You may download a copy of the Work on one occasion to one personal computer (including tablet, laptop, desktop, or other such devices). You may make one back-up copy of the Work to avoid losing it.
3. The unauthorised use or distribution of copyrighted or other proprietary content is illegal and could subject you to liability for substantial money damages. You will be liable for any damage resulting from your misuse of the Work or any violation of this License Agreement, including any infringement by you of copyrights or proprietary rights.

Disclaimer:

Bentham Science Publishers does not guarantee that the information in the Work is error-free, or warrant that it will meet your requirements or that access to the Work will be uninterrupted or error-free. The Work is provided "as is" without warranty of any kind, either express or implied or statutory, including, without limitation, implied warranties of merchantability and fitness for a particular purpose. The entire risk as to the results and performance of the Work is assumed by you. No responsibility is assumed by Bentham Science Publishers, its staff, editors and/or authors for any injury and/or damage to persons or property as a matter of products liability, negligence or otherwise, or from any use or operation of any methods, products instruction, advertisements or ideas contained in the Work.

Limitation of Liability:

In no event will Bentham Science Publishers, its staff, editors and/or authors, be liable for any damages, including, without limitation, special, incidental and/or consequential damages and/or damages for lost data and/or profits arising out of (whether directly or indirectly) the use or inability to use the Work. The entire liability of Bentham Science Publishers shall be limited to the amount actually paid by you for the Work.

General:

1. Any dispute or claim arising out of or in connection with this License Agreement or the Work (including non-contractual disputes or claims) will be governed by and construed in accordance with the laws of the U.A.E. as applied in the Emirate of Dubai. Each party agrees that the courts of the Emirate of Dubai shall have exclusive jurisdiction to settle any dispute or claim arising out of or in connection with this License Agreement or the Work (including non-contractual disputes or claims).
2. Your rights under this License Agreement will automatically terminate without notice and without the

need for a court order if at any point you breach any terms of this License Agreement. In no event will any delay or failure by Bentham Science Publishers in enforcing your compliance with this License Agreement constitute a waiver of any of its rights.

3. You acknowledge that you have read this License Agreement, and agree to be bound by its terms and conditions. To the extent that any other terms and conditions presented on any website of Bentham Science Publishers conflict with, or are inconsistent with, the terms and conditions set out in this License Agreement, you acknowledge that the terms and conditions set out in this License Agreement shall prevail.

Bentham Science Publishers Ltd.
Executive Suite Y - 2
PO Box 7917, Saif Zone
Sharjah, U.A.E.
Email: subscriptions@benthamscience.net

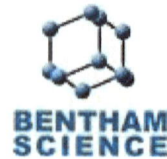

BENTHAM
SCIENCE

CONTENTS

FOREWORD

This book is an innovative and up-to-date addition to the literature on heart failure in children. It is written by some of the most prestigious paediatric cardiologists. The various chapters describe the clinical picture as well as the role of imaging, interventional cardiology and surgery in the diagnosis and management of heart failure in infants and children. One chapter also highlight hypertrophic cardiomyopathy in pediatric population. The text is easy to read and facilitates the understanding of the most complex aspects of heart failure.

This book will be welcomed by trainees and experienced pediatric cardiologists as well as established heart surgeons and intensivists.

Alain Fraisse
Royal Brompton & Harefield Hospital Trust
London
U.K.

PREFACE

The first Edition of *"Heart Failure in Pediatric Patients"*: *A Textbook of Pediatric Heart Failure,* serves as a core learning tool designed to help cardiologists, pediatricians, pediatric nurses and students at all levels, from trainees to highly specialized practitioners, confront the challenge of staying abreast of this evolving field.

The field of heart failure in pediatric populations has perhaps recently initiated more registries and clinical trials than previously. This age group has special concerns and particularities regarding their clinical picture and management. Therefore, multiple disciplines have been involved in the management of heart failure in this age group.

In this edition, we tried to answer all the questions concerning this field, and be up-to-date in all our resources.

This e-book was prepared by a group of eminent international specialists from different international centers. All of them are experts in one of the related fields.

We tried to make this edition an informative source of practical utility; to help readers surmount the swift change in heart failure knowledge.

Within chapters, you will notice the novelty and the adherence to the guidelines as well as the experience aspect of the authors.

This book contains very interesting images as well as videos that illustrate and accurately describe cases regarding the field of pediatric heart failure.

After reading this book, you will be able to deal with heart failure in this special entity of pediatric populations in different age groups.

This book contains various key components of the *"Heart Failure in Pediatric Patients"*, assembled in a personalized way to meet the needs of each practitioner.

In this e-book, we described the pathophysiology, classification and clinical data of heart failure with special concern in pediatric populations. We emphasized on a special group of infants with congenital heart disease with all aspects concerning their diagnosis and management.

We displayed different modes of imaging diagnosis for heart failure and then concentrated on one of the most important investigations as myocardial biopsy.

In this book, we described the detailed radiological and imaging investigations for heart failure in general; however we spoke about the investigation of certain pediatric and congenital heart disease within the chapters. The intent was to broaden the scope of target audience and help the readers to discover all about the field of heart failure investigations.

We described one of the most important pathological types of heart failure; hypertrophic cardiomyopathy. We put this topic in a separate chapter due to its special importance.

We described the modes of management of heart failure in pediatric patients. Finally, we presented the surgical management of terminal cases of heart failure in pediatric age groups.

We hope that readers will find *"Heart Failure in Pediatric Patients"* and its associated learning tools useful in their quest to stay abreast of this ever-evolving field.

Mohammad El Tahlawi
Zagazig University Hospitals,
Cardiology Department,
University St,
Zagazig,
Egypt

List of Contributors

Ahmed Aljizeeri   King Abdulaziz Cardiac Center, King Abdulaziz Medical City-Riyadh, Riyadh, Kingdom of Saudi Arabia

Ahmed A Alsaileek   King Abdulaziz Cardiac Center, King Abdulaziz Medical City-Riyadh, Riyadh, Kingdom of Saudi Arabia

Anas Taqatqa   Rush University Medical Center, Chicago, USA

Kasey J. Chaszczewski   Rush University Medical Center, Chicago, USA

Khaled Abdelhady   Rush University Medical Center, Chicago, USA

Mohammad El Tahlawi   Rush University Medical Center, Chicago, USA
Department of Ocean Studies and Marine Biology, Zagazig University Hospital, Zagazig, Egypt
Cardiology Department, National Heart Institute, Giza, Egypt
Inherited Cardiomyopathy Clinical and Research Unit, Magdi Yacoub Heart Foundation, Cairo, Egypt

Mouaz H. Al-Mallah   King Abdulaziz Cardiac Center, King Abdulaziz Medical City-Riyadh, Riyadh, Kingdom of Saudi Arabia

Pimpak Prachasilchai   Evelina London Children's Hospital, London, UK

Ralf J. Holzer   Weill Cornell Medicine, NewYork-Presbyterian Komansky Children's Hospital, USA

Shakeel Ahmed Qureshi   Evelina London Children's Hospital, London, UK

Sawsan Awad   Medical Center, Rush University, Chicago, USA

Sarah Moharem Elgamal   Cardiology Department, National Heart Institute, Giza, Egypt

Shehab M. Anwer   Cardiology Department, National Heart Institute, Giza, Egypt

Ziyad M. Hijazi   Sidra Medical and Research Center, Doha, Qatar

Heart Failure in Pediatric Patients

Pimpak Prachasilchai[1], Mohammad El Tahlawi[2] and Shakeel Ahmed Qureshi[1,*]

[1] *Evelina London Children's Hospital, London, UK*

[2] *Zagazig University Hospital, Zagazig, Egypt*

Abstract: The diagnosis of heart failure in children remains challenging. It precipitates changes in circulatory abnormalities, multiple cellular processes and neuro-hormonal status. Many cases are due to congenital disorders .Clinical picture in children ranges from being asymptomatic to having severe life-threatening symptoms. Ross classification was originally developed to determine the presence and severity of heart failure in infants and younger children. Non-invasive imaging studies are necessary in order to make the diagnosis of heart failure in children. Management ranges from medical, interventional to surgical procedures. Heart transplantation remains an acceptable treatment for children with end-stage heart failure.

Keywords: Cardiomyopathy, Congenital Heart, Echocardiography, Heart Transplantation, Heart Failure, Inotropes, Mechanical Circulatory Support, Pulmonary Blood Flow, Ross Classification.

INTRODUCTION

The diagnosis of heart failure in children remains challenging compared with adults. This is due to various manifestations from the wide variety of cardiac aetiologies, clinical onsets and aspects of its pathophysiology. There are no standard guidelines for paediatric heart failure; however, heart failure occurs in children with congenital malformations, which may be associated with both underlying congenital heart diseases (CHD) with preserved systolic function, and/or myocardial dysfunction.

Heart failure is a clinical condition in which the heart pumps insufficient blood to meet the metabolic demands of the organs due to poor contractility or excessive preload and afterload. The components – such as history, characteristic signs and symptoms, and diagnostic tools (including echocardiography, exercise testing,

---

* **Corresponding author Shakeel A. Qureshi:** Evelina London Children's Hospital, Westminster Bridge Road, London SE1 7EH, UK; Tel: 00442071884547; Fax: 00442071884556; E-mail: Shakeel.Qureshi@gstt.nhs.uk

Mohammad El Tahlawi (Ed.)
All rights reserved-© 2020 Bentham Science Publishers

biomarkers and cardiac catheterisation) – can provide the information necessary for proper diagnosis and treatment, leading, in turn, to a reduced mortality rate.

Pathophysiology

Heart failure precipitates changes in circulatory abnormalities, multiple cellular processes and neuro-hormonal status. These changes serve as compensatory mechanisms to help maintain cardiac output (CO), primarily by the Frank-Starling mechanism and arterial blood pressure by systemic vasoconstriction. Most heart failure therapy involves counteracting elevated systemic and pulmonary vascular resistances that accompany neuro-humoral abnormalities, including increased sympathetic tone and activation of the renin-angiotensin-aldosterone system. These mechanisms not only have an impact on the manifestation of heart failure in children, but are also essential for the development of pharmacologic intervention.

There are two main compensatory processes of heart failure, namely, circulatory compensation and neuro-hormonal activation (Table **1**).

Table 1. Compensatory mechanisms of heart failure.

Circulatory Compensation	Neurohormonal Activation
Frank-Starling mechanism	Renin-angiotensin-aldosterone system
Ventricular remodeling	Antidiuretic hormone (Vasopressin)
Tachycardia	Sympathetic nervous system
	Catecholamine
	Endothelins
	Natriuretic peptides

Circulatory Compensation

The Frank-Starling mechanism Fig. (**1**) describes the changes in preload and cardiac output (CO). In heart failure, an increase in the venous return stretches the ventricular wall, causing the cardiac muscle to contract more forcefully, thereby resulting in an increase in stoke volume (SV) in order to maintain CO. There are some limitations of this mechanism in the fetus and infants, presumably due to myocardial immaturity.

Another important compensatory mechanism is ventricular remodelling, such as more spherical, dilatation and hypertrophy, in order to maintain CO. However, the ventricular hypertrophy may lead to diastolic dysfunction. Reduced CO with hypotension activates arterial baroreflexes, increasing the sympathetic tone whilst decreasing parasympathetic tone. This results in an increased heart rate and myocardial contractility. Catecholamine released during heart failure also causes tachycardia.

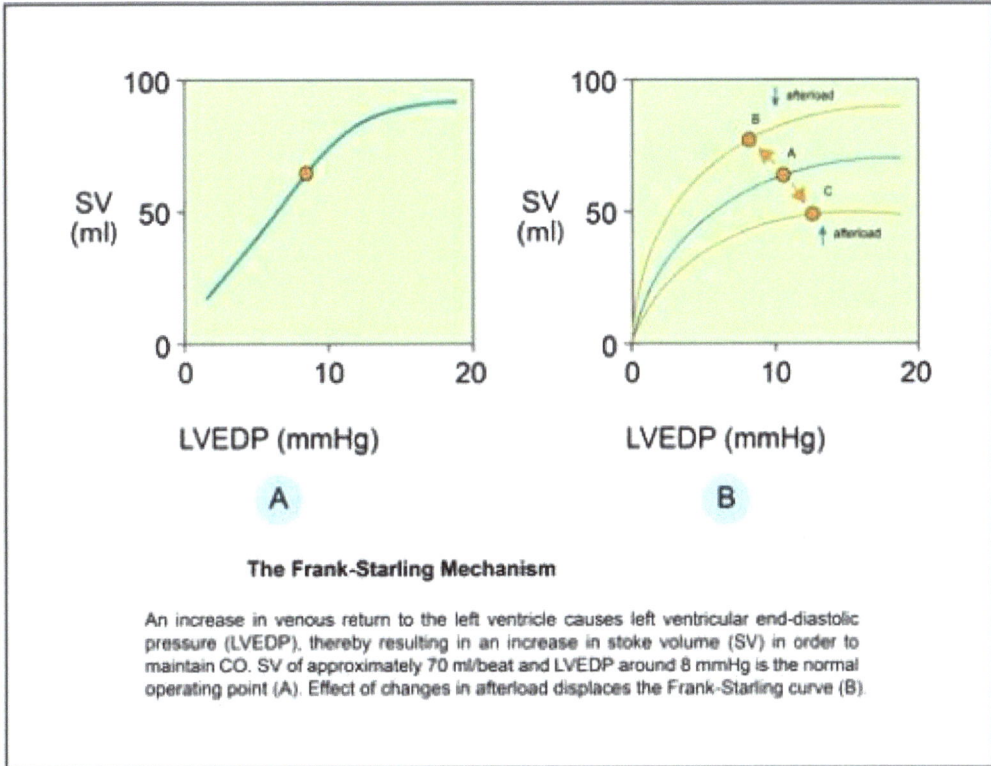

The Frank-Starling Mechanism

An increase in venous return to the left ventricle causes left ventricular end-diastolic pressure (LVEDP), thereby resulting in an increase in stoke volume (SV) in order to maintain CO. SV of approximately 70 ml/beat and LVEDP around 8 mmHg is the normal operating point (A). Effect of changes in afterload displaces the Frank-Starling curve (B).

Fig. (1). Frank Starling Mechanism.

Neurohormonal Activation

The renin-angiotensin-aldosterone system regulates the systemic blood pressure and the fluid balance in the body. Stimulation of the renin-angiotensin-aldosterone system is activated by hypoperfusion, leading to increased concentrations of renin, angiotensin II, and aldosterone. When renal blood flow is reduced, juxtaglomerular cells lining the afferent arterioles in the kidneys secrete renin before catalyzing the protein angiotensinogen, produced in the liver, into angiotensin I. This is then converted by angiotensin-converting enzyme (ACE), which is released from the lung capillaries, into angiotensin II, which stimulates aldosterone secretion *via* receptors in the zona glomerulosa in the adrenal cortex of the adrenal gland. Aldosterone causes more tubular salt and water reabsorption, and more potassium excretion, which leads to an increase in preload and CO (Fig. **2**). Angiotensin II also stimulates the posterior pituitary gland to secrete antidiuretic hormone (ADH) – also known as vasopressin. This acts on two receptors, causing vasoconstriction and an increase in the reabsorption of water, which promotes more water retention and hyponatremia. Angiotensin II is also a powerful arteriolar vasoconstrictor throughout the body and stimulates the sympathetic nervous system through actions on both central and peripheral sites. This leads to an increase in the venous and arterial tones and in plasma noradrenaline levels, resulting in the progressive retention of salt and water. In addition, norepinephrine in chronic heart failure has important effects on cardiac myocyte necrosis and cell death by apoptosis.

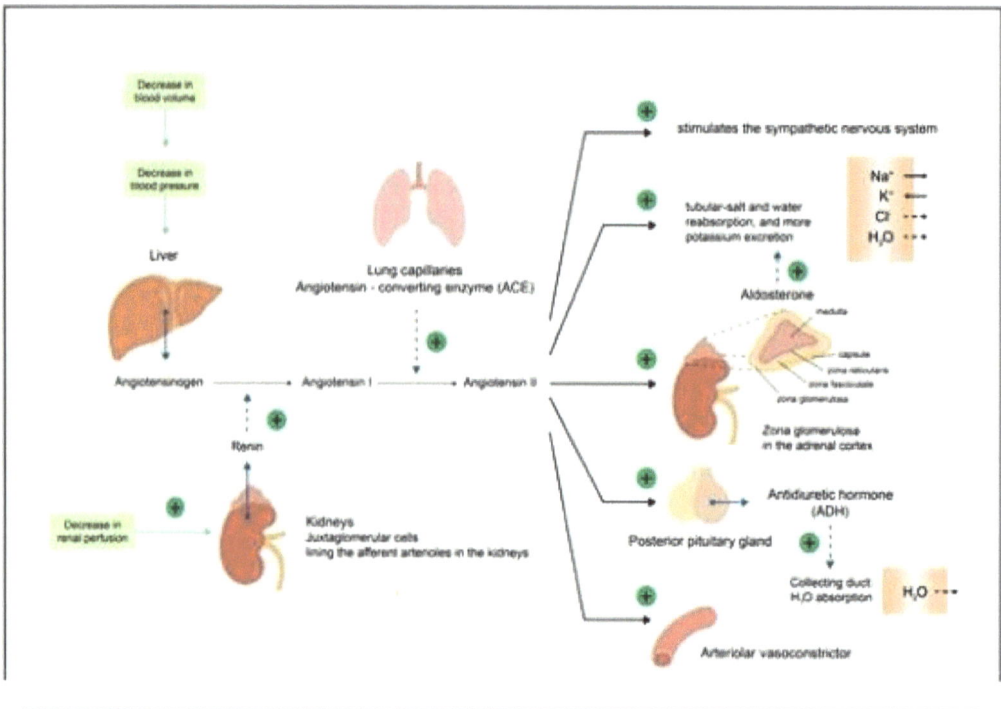

Fig. (2). The Renin-angiotensin aldosterone System.

Endothelin-1 (ET-1) is released by the endothelium, and angiotensin II is a powerful activator of ET-1 gene expression. It is a potent vasoconstrictor peptide. The plasma ET-1 level is increased in heart failure patients and is correlated with the severity of pulmonary hypertension, the prognosis of heart failure and the mortality rate.

Two types of natriuretic peptides are released from the heart: atrial natriuretic peptide (ANP) and brain natriuretic peptide (BNP). The former is released from the atrium due to the stretching of the atrial wall. The action of this hormone includes vasodilation, diuresis and natriuresis. BNP is also released from the heart, predominantly from the ventricles, with similar actions to ANP. Both act as antagonists to the effects of angiotensin II on the vascular tone, aldosterone secretion and salt reabsorption. They are important mediators for diagnosing and assessing the prognosis of heart failure, shown in many studies [1 - 4].

In the embryo, the parallel circulation has a compensatory nature, making most of the congenital cardiac anomalies well tolerated. However, heart failure can occur in utero due to high venous pressure in case of cardiomyopathy, marked tachycardia, severe valve regurgitation and other high output states [5].

Clinical Presentations

Children with heart failure often have non-specific signs and symptoms, particularly neonates and infants. In addition, there are many types of congenital heart defects, from simple to complex, and these range from being asymptomatic to having severe life-threatening symptoms.

Congenital heart defects (CHD) are the most common type of birth defect. They affect eight out of every thousand new-borns. Approximately 70% of cases of CHD are diagnosed in the first year of life, and heart failure associated with CHD occurs in about 20% of all CHD patients [6]. The causes of heart failure include dilated cardiomyopathy, which is supported by the data from the UK, which indicates that the incidence of heart failure assessed at first presentation to a hospital is around 0.87 per 100,000 [7].

There is also a much higher proportion of children with heart failure, who have undergone cardiac procedures (61.4%) compared with adults (0.28%). This reflects the incidence of CHD, the frequent surgical intervention to correct the defects, and the subsequent and eventual deterioration in cardiac function observed in many of these paediatric patients [8]. Despite receiving appropriate surgical intervention, as many as 20% of children born with CHD will eventually have chronic failure.

Presentation of heart failure varies with the age of the child [9]. Signs of the congestion in an infant generally include irritability, grunting, tachypnea, difficulty with feeding, and failure to thrive. Often, they have diaphoresis during feedings, which is possibly related to the catecholamine release that occurs, when they are feeding while in respiratory distress (Table **2**). Older children may have more specific features, such as fatigue, exercise intolerance, breathlessness, and/or evidence of pulmonary congestion. Decompensated heart failure is characterized by signs and symptoms of low cardiac output, which may be followed by signs of renal and hepatic failure.

Table 2. Signs and symptoms of heart failure.

Signs and symptoms of heart failure	
Increased sympathetic activity	**Systemic and venous congestion**
Irritability	Cardiomegaly
Diaphoresis	Hepatomegaly
Tachycardia	Tachypnoea
Oliguria	Wheezing (cardiac asthma)
Cool extremities	Jugular venous distension
	Extremity oedema/ascites/pleural effusion.

Classifications of Heart Failure

There are several classifications. The Ross classification was originally developed to determine the presence and severity of heart failure in infants and younger children [10, 11]. It has subsequently been modified for all paediatric ages, incorporating feeding difficulties, growth problems and symptoms of exercise intolerance into a numeric score comparable with the New York Heart Association (NYHA) classification for adults (Table **3**). The NYHA classification [12] is used worldwide, particularly for adults, and focuses on the limitations of exercise capacity and the symptomatic status of the disease. The American College of Cardiology Foundation (ACCF) and the American Heart Association (AHA) stages of heart failure recognize that both risk factors and abnormalities of cardiac structure are associated with heart failure Table **4** [13].

Table 3. Ross classification for children [9].

Class	Interpretation
I	No limitations or symptoms.
II	Mild tachypnoea or diaphoresis with feeding in infants. Dyspnoea on exertion in older children; no growth failure.
III	Marked tachypnoea or diaphoresis with feeding or exertion and prolonged feeding times with growth failure from heart failure.
IV	Symptomatic at rest with tachypnoea, retraction, grunting, or diaphoresis.

The New York University Paediatric Heart Failure Index (NYU PHFI) was introduced to assess the severity of heart failure in paediatric patients by using scoring based on physiological indicators and medical therapy, which were correlated with electrocardiographic, echocardiographic and biochemical markers better than the Ross and NYHA scoring systems in children with a homogeneous type of heart disease [14, 15].

Table 4. Comparison of ACCF/AHA Stages and NYHA Functional Classifications [12].

ACCF/AHA Stages of heart failure			NYHA Functional Classification
A	At high risk for heart failure but without structural heart disease or symptoms of heart failure.	None	
B	Structural heart disease but without signs or symptoms of heart failure.	I	No limitation of physical activity. Ordinary physical activity does not cause symptoms of heart failure.
C	Structural heart disease with prior or current symptoms of heart failure.	I	No limitation of physical activity. Ordinary physical activity does not cause symptoms of heart failure.
		II	Slight limitation of physical activity. Comfortable at rest, but ordinary physical activity results in symptoms of heart failure.
		III	Marked limitation of physical activity. Comfortable at rest, but less than ordinary activity causes symptoms of heart failure.
		IV	Unable to carry out any physical activity without symptoms of heart failure, or symptoms of heart failure at rest.
D	Refractory HF requiring specialized interventions.	IV	Unable to carry out any physical activity without symptoms of heart failure, or symptoms of heart failure at rest.

(ACCF: American College of Cardiology Foundation, AHA: American Heart Association, and NYHA: New York Heart Association)

Aetiology

The aetiologies for heart failure in children are significantly different from adults. Many cases are due to congenital disorders, which mainly result from volume or pressure overload (Table **5**). They subsequently suffer from high-output cardiac failure or chronic volume overload associated with valvar insufficiency. Another significant cause of heart failure in children is cardiomyopathy, which leads to low-output cardiac failure.

Table 5. Congenital related aetiologies of heart failure in children.

Excessive pulmonary blood flow
Left-to-right shunt: ventricular septal defect, patent ductus arteriosus, atrioventricular septal defect, coronary artery fistula.
Pressure overload
Left sided obstruction: coarctation of the aorta, severe aortic stenosis.

(Table 5) cont.....

Excessive pulmonary blood flow
Right sided obstruction: critical pulmonary stenosis, pulmonary atresia.
Valvar insufficiency
Atrioventricular valve or semilunar valve insufficiency: Ebstein's anomaly, aortic valve insufficiency due to a bicuspid aortic valve, pulmonary insufficiency following tetralogy of Fallot repair.
Complex congenital heart disease
Single ventricles: hypoplastic left heart syndrome, tricuspid atresia.
Cardiomyopathy
Anomalous left coronary artery from the pulmonary artery (ALCAPA).
Idiopathic.
Mitochondrial or genetic disorders.
Abnormalities in fatty acid, amino acid, glycogen, and mucopolysaccharide metabolism.

Excessive Pulmonary Blood Flow

In conditions with left-to-right shunt, blood from the systemic arterial circulation mixes with the systemic venous blood. Significant left-to-right shunts may cause congestive heart failure symptoms despite normal systolic ventricular function. Pulmonary over-circulation secondary to left-to-right shunt commonly causes heart failure in early infancy. The most common defect is a ventricular septal defect (VSD) that presents around 6-8 weeks of age as the pulmonary vascular resistance falls. Other left-to-right shunts, including complex congenital heart disease with unrestricted pulmonary blood flow, present similarly. Among the group of left-to-right shunts, atrial septal defects (ASD) almost never lead to congestive failure in infancy and very rarely in childhood. The clinical presentation of patients with an atrioventricular septal defect depends on the magnitude of blood flow through the VSD and the addition of atrioventricular valve regurgitation. Patients with mild valve regurgitation may be asymptomatic early in life, and therefore difficult to diagnose, before developing cyanosis from advanced pulmonary vascular disease. The haemodynamics of coronary artery fistulas depend on the resistance of the fistulous connection, the site of fistula termination, the size of the communication and the potential for development of myocardial ischemia.

Pressure Overload

Left Sided Obstruction

Congenital left-sided cardiac lesions can precipitate heart failure due to abnormal afterload on the left ventricle, resulting in ventricular hypertrophy, increased oxygen demand and subendocardial ischaemia, and increasing pulmonary venous pressure with a predisposition to pulmonary oedema. Severe, left-sided heart obstruction may also lead to inadequate blood flow to the organs of the body, causing profound shock, necrotising enterocolitis (NEC) and sepsis, particularly in infancy. Myocardial function often improves in these infants following relief of the obstruction.

Right-Sided Obstruction

Isolated pulmonary valve stenosis represents 80-90% of pulmonary stenosis cases. Patients with severe pulmonary stenosis cause suprasystemic right ventricular pressure, leading to congestive failure in early life, needing early intervention. If these patients have an associated ASD, right-to-left shunting may occur, resulting in cyanosis.

Rarely, children with pulmonary atresia with VSD, who have significant major aortopulmonary collateral arteries (MAPCAs), may have excessive pulmonary blood flow, and then develop symptoms of congestive heart failure. The development of congestive failure in tetralogy of Fallot (TOF) may rarely occur, but then it is usually associated with bacterial endocarditis and severe anaemia.

Valvar Insufficiency

Both atrioventricular and semilunar valve regurgitation are significant causes of heart failure due to left ventricular volume overload, particularly in cases of congenital heart defects, for instance Ebstein's anomaly, aortic valve insufficiency due to a bicuspid aortic valve, and pulmonary insufficiency following TOF repair. The severity of heart failure depends on the degree of valvar regurgitation. Patients with clinically significant valve regurgitation may develop signs of heart failure.

Neonates with Ebstein's anomaly may present with heart failure resulting from severe tricuspid regurgitation, abnormal right ventricular geometry, and hypoxia because of right-to-left atrial shunting. Bicuspid aortic valve disease is one of the most common congenital heart defects, causing either aortic valve stenosis or insufficiency or both. Aortic valve insufficiency occurs in around 12% of patients, and it leads to left ventricular volume overload and an increase in the stroke volume [16]. The progression of left ventricular enlargement may occur, and may produce subendocardial and myocardial ischaemia. There are some associated anomalies, such as coarctation of the aorta or interrupted aortic arch, which result in an increase in the diastolic flow of blood into the left ventricle. The surgical approach to the relief of severe pulmonary stenosis in TOF includes patch augmentation of the right ventricular outflow tract and resection of pulmonary valve, causing pulmonary regurgitation, this progressive pulmonary regurgitation results in progressive dilatation of the right ventricle and an increase in the end-diastolic volume, leading to a deterioration of the systolic function.

Complex Congenital Heart Disease

The assessment of the heart failure in single-ventricle patients is very complicated. The clinical symptoms depend on the degree of obstruction of the outflow and inflow, the severity of the atrioventricular valve regurgitation, and the geometry of the systemic ventricle.

Hypoplastic left heart syndrome with mitral valve atresia and restrictive ASD is physiologically the same as pulmonary venous obstruction, causing pulmonary venous congestion. Tricuspid atresia with restrictive ASD leads to systemic venous obstruction. Conduction disturbances and arrhythmias may also cause ventricular dysfunction in these patients. Fontan operation is mainly used to reduce the volume load on the systemic ventricle, resulting in a reduction in the ventricular size and hypertrophy [17, 18].

Cardiomyopathy

An anomalous left coronary artery from the pulmonary artery (ALCAPA) may cause heart failure due to the retrograde flow from the left coronary artery into the pulmonary artery, resulting in myocardial ischaemia. Some patients may present with mitral valve regurgitation due to papillary muscle infarction, which is usually resolved after surgical relocation of the coronary artery [19 - 21].

Although cardiomyopathy is relatively rare, nearly half of the children who develop heart failure undergo transplantation or die within several years [22]. Dilated cardiomyopathy (DCM) is the most common type of cardiomyopathy, and it is usually diagnosed in children aged less than one year [22 - 24]. DCM has a wide variety of aetiologies, such as idiopathic, mitochondrial or genetic disorders, and abnormalities in fatty acids, amino acids, glycogen or the mucopolysaccharide metabolism [25 - 27].

Investigations

Non-invasive imaging studies are necessary in order to make the diagnosis of heart failure in children. A chest radiograph is useful for determining the severity of cardiomegaly and pulmonary oedema. In addition, it helps to identify whether it is the heart or the lung condition that is worsening the patients' symptoms. An electrocardiogram (ECG) is also a non-invasive investigation, which can show the chamber enlargement, ventricular hypertrophy and rhythm disorders. However, advanced cardiac imaging, such as an echocardiogram and/or cardiac magnetic resonance imaging (CMRI), is required.

Echocardiography remains the most frequently used imaging modality. It is very useful for determining the cause of heart failure in terms of both its structural and functional details, particularly in the case of congenital heart defects, including abnormal myocardium. This investigation can also assess the left ventricular ejection fraction and other measurements of the pumping function, and it can take into account variations in age and body size [28]. A poor ventricular ejection fraction and fractional shortening are correlated with a poor outcome in children with DCM [7, 29]. However, the assessment of the right ventricle and a single ventricle remains complicated due to their geometry. The Doppler myocardial performance index is very useful for functional assessment in complex heart disease, particularly of the systemic right ventricle [30]. Three-dimensional (3D) echocardiography is also useful for identifying additional structural defects, especially in the valves.

Although an exercise stress test cannot be performed in infants and young children, it is helpful in older children and adults with congenital heart defects. Deteriorations in performance during serial exercise testing are used as an indication for intervention in some congenital heart diseases, such as the timing of a pulmonary valve replacement in pulmonary insufficiency following TOF repair, and occasionally for the timing of intervention in aortic valve stenosis patients [31].

Cardiovascular magnetic resonance (CMR) has a role in the diagnosis and management of congenital heart diseases in providing haemodynamic data and information on the intracardiac anatomy, which used to be obtained *via* cardiac catheterisation [32 - 34]. For instance, the great vessels, the systemic and pulmonary veins, shunts, and the vascular and valvar flow can be assessed by CMR [35, 36]. CMR can accurately assess the right ventricular and single ventricular function in complex defects and allows reconstruction in any imaging plane, providing complete assessment [37]. Myocardial inflammation, myocardial scarring and fibrosis are regarded as common pathologies in cardiomyopathies. They play a major role in determining whether the myocardium scarring is reversible or not, and the aetiology of a DCM, both of which can be assessed by CMR [38 - 41]. However, there are some limitations of CMRs, such as technical difficulties, particularly with critical patients who are unstable. In addition, small anatomical structures may not be visualized clearly, and cardiac catheterization may be required to identify lesions, especially in patients, who need therapeutic cardiac intervention, which can be performed at the same time.

Biomarkers are increasingly being used as a diagnostic tool and as an outcome predictor in the treatment of adults with heart failure. However, in children, there are no guidelines for the use of brain natriuretic peptide (BNP) and N-terminal pro-BNP levels, as is the case with adults [42]. One study showed that a BNP level of more than 140 pg/mL in stable paediatric outpatients with mild-t--moderate heart failure symptoms can be used to identify children at the risk of hospitalization for worsening symptoms, death, or transplantation [43, 44].

Genetic testing and counselling have also become increasingly important in the diagnosis and management of heart failure in patients, who are diagnosed with DCM [45].

In conclusion, the assessment for heart failure related with congenital heart diseases involves a variety of investigations in order to minimize harm and increase accuracy.

Treatment

The management of heart failure in children with congenital heart disease is difficult and challenging due to the differences in the physiology and pharmacokinetics of neonates, infants and older children.

Congestive Heart Failure in the Neonate and Infant

Identification of the aetiology plays a major role in the management of heart failure in newborns or infants, which can arise from non-cardiac or cardiac aetiologies. The former include sepsis, hypoxaemia, hydrops and persistent pulmonary hypertension, particularly in acute onset cases. The children frequently develop acidaemia, respiratory compromise or failure, and metabolic derangements (such as hypoglycaemia, hypocalcaemia or hypomagnesaemia), all of which require early recognition and urgent therapy.

Congenital heart defects (especially in neonates with duct-dependent lesions), large left-to-right shunt lesions, myocardial abnormalities or arrhythmias lead to acute onset of heart failure. The management of such patients aims to reduce symptoms, correct metabolic abnormalities and maintain haemodynamics.

Patients with duct-dependent lesions – such as coarctation of the aorta, hypoplastic left heart syndrome, aortic valve disease, pulmonary valve stenosis or pulmonary valve atresia – need **Prostaglandin E1 (PGE1)**. As the main effect of this medication is to maintain the patency of, or to reopen, the ductus arteriosus, echocardiography should be performed before its administration. If echocardiography is not immediately available, prostaglandin can be infused in order to save the lives of the newborns or infants. The recommended starting dose of PGE1 is 0.05-0.1 mcg/kg/min, which can be titrated up to 0.4 mcg/kg/min, depending on clinical signs, oxygen saturation and arterial blood gas [46]. The maintenance dose can be reduced to 0.002-0.05 mcg/kg/min [47].

Medical therapy in infants with heart failure due to systemic and pulmonary vascular congestion mainly consists of **diuretics**, especially intravenous diuretics, such as loop diuretics for the initial treatment. Non-pharmacological measures, such as fluid restriction, should be considered until the infants are established on oral diuretics and tolerating feeds well. Continuous infusion of a loop diuretic should also be considered if patients fail to respond to intermittent administration. Monitoring of side-effects for electrolyte disturbances, renal insufficiency and hypotension, is necessary. In addition, long-term administration in neonates may cause sensorineural hearing loss [48]. **Digoxin** is a cardiac glycoside that acts *via* the inhibition of the Na^+, K^+-ATPase pump. Studies have shown unclear results as to the role of digoxin in heart failure due to volume overload conditions [49, 50].

Newborns with low cardiac output should be considered for the administration of a catecholamine, such as dopamine, dobutamine or epinephrine, in order to maintain haemodynamics and improve end-organ function. Neonates require a greater plasma concentration of exogenous catecholamine to affect the same increase in cardiac output and blood pressure as in older children, because neonates have a larger volume distribution and higher clearance, leading to the low efficacy of catecholamines [51, 52]. **Dopamine** is a sympathomimetic that stimulates beta-adrenergic receptors, as well as alpha-adrenergic receptors and dopaminergic receptors, causing increased contractility and heart rate, peripheral vasoconstriction, vasodilation or augmented renal blood flow, which relate to the dose. Common side effects include tachycardia, increased myocardial oxygen consumption and arrhythmias. **Dobutamine** stimulates the beta-adrenergic receptors in the myocardium and the peripheral vasculature, causing increased myocardial contractility and decreased peripheral and pulmonary vascular tone [53]. **Epinephrine** can be used in life-threatening situations, in which it can increase blood pressure, heart rate and contractility, but it leads to ischaemia, atrial or ventricular arrhythmias, and increased myocardial oxygen consumption.

Milrinone is a phosphodiesterase inhibitor (PDEI) that acts by increasing cyclic adenosine monophosphate (cAMP), thereby providing similar effects to inotropic drugs except with additional afterload reduction. Milrinone is also a vasodilator in systemic and pulmonary vascular beds, which is very useful in neonates with low cardiac output syndrome in the immediate postoperative period [54]. Moreover, it does not interact with beta receptors, making it less likely to cause tachycardia than other inotropic agents.

Angiotensin-converting enzyme inhibitors (ACEI), such as captopril and enalapril, can improve cardiac output by reducing the systemic vascular resistance, leading to an improvement in the symptoms and haemodynamic status [55, 56]. However, this has some risks in neonates because it mainly affects glomerular infiltration, so close monitoring and low dose administration should be considered.

A **calcium chloride** infusion may also support the blood pressure and increase contractility when ionized calcium concentrations are low. **Oxygen and hyperventilation** are helpful to reduce the pulmonary vascular resistance. However, as the goal of treatment in duct-dependent systemic blood flow is to achieve a pulmonary to systemic circulation flow ratio of 1:1, an oxygen saturation of 75% to 80% may be desirable. The correction of electrolyte imbalance and optimization of nutrition are also important for this group of patients. Nutritional supplements should be considered to ensure that patients receive enough calories to compensate for the increased energy requirements resulting from heart diseases.

The curative therapy is directed towards the cause of heart failure. Infants with left-to-right shunt lesions who have significant symptoms, especially failure to thrive, or who fail to respond to medication, should undergo surgical closure of the underlying defect in order to minimize the risk of pulmonary vascular disease. However, patients with unrestrictive VSD who grow normally should be observed. If the VSD remains unrestrictive, most of them should undergo surgical closure at the age of 3-6 months. In the neonates, critical aortic valve stenosis and pulmonary valve stenosis can be treated by balloon valvoplasty. In symptomatic newborns with aortic coarctation, surgical repair is usually performed on an urgent basis following initial stabilization. Palliative procedures, such as the Blalock-Taussig shunt, the Glenn procedure and the Norwood procedure, can often be used to stabilize infants with ductal-dependent systemic or pulmonary blood flow lesions.

Congestive Heart Failure in the Older Children

Excessive Pulmonary Blood Flow

The mainstays of medical therapy have historically been **digitalis** and **diuretics**. The use of digitalis for neonates, infants and older children with heart failure is still controversial. However, **loop diuretics**, such as furosemide, have been shown to improve clinical symptoms on a background of digitalis administration [57]. In addition, furosemide can decrease pulmonary congestion and heart failure symptoms. The dose of digoxin is 0.005-0.010 mg/kg/day orally, divided into twice daily doses, and not to exceed 0.125-0.25 mg. However, the dose may need to be decreased in the presence of signs of toxicity, for instance, confusion, poor appetite, nausea, vomiting, diarrhoea and palpitations. The addition of **spironolactone** (aldosterone antagonists) at low doses (25 mg/day), shows significant decreases in both morbidity and death in adults [58]. This medication may be indicated in patients with diuretic-induced hypokalaemia. The usual dosage for children of spironolactone is 1-3.3 mg/kg/day in single or divided doses. For more severe congestive heart failure, hydrochlorothiazide or metolazone may be added in order to achieve a synergistic effect. Afterload reduction with **ACEI**, in paediatric patients with left-to-right shunt lesions may improve growth, as has been seen in some children [59, 60]. On the other hand, unwanted effects, such as renal failure or a severe cough, may develop [61]. Because ACEI and spironolactone cause potassium retention, the potassium level should be monitored regularly. There is no efficacy data on **angiotensin receptor blocker** (ARB), such as candesartan, losartan and valsartan, in children with heart failure. They should only be used in patients with intolerance to ACEI, which is in line with the general practice for adults [62]. After infancy, children with a moderate-sized VSD or PDA, who develop left-sided heart dilation, indicating left-ventricular volume overload, are a class I indication for undergoing surgical or percutaneous closure [63]. Half of the deaths of inpatients with untreated PDA involve endocarditis, and these patients have a strong indication for curative treatment.

Pressure Overload

Severe valvar stenosis can lead to ventricular hypertrophy or ventricular dysfunction; however, ventricular function improves and usually normalizes after balloon valvoplasty or surgery [64, 65]. The indication for aortic balloon valvoplasty in isolated cases is a peak-to-peak systolic pressure gradient across the aortic valve at rest higher than 50 mmHg (by catheter), or a gradient (by catheter) of more than 40 mmHg if there are clinical symptoms, such as angina or syncope, or the presence of electrocardiographic ST-T wave changes [66]. Higher aortic valve gradients increase the risk of sudden death, and there is an increased risk of serious arrhythmias [67]. Afterload reduction using an ACEI is indicated in the presence of left ventricular dysfunction, regardless of symptoms. A pulmonary valvoplasty is indicated for patients who have a peak-to-peak catheter gradient or echocardiographic peak instantaneous gradient of more than 40 mmHg, with symptoms or RV dysfunction [66]. Unfortunately, residual stenosis and the occurrence of valvar regurgitation are the main complications [68, 69].

Coarctation may also cause heart failure. However, older children may have minimal symptoms due to collateral development. Coarctation repair is typically planned electively, and coarctation stenting can be considered, depending on the anatomy. Medications might be used to control blood pressure before surgery. Although repairing aortic coarctation improves blood pressure, many patients still need to take antihypertensive drugs due to persistent hypertension.

Valvar Insufficiency

Medical treatment for this group of patients is similar to those with excessive pulmonary blood flow due to having the same physiology (volume overload). It includes diuretics, digoxin and ACEI. Ebstein's anomaly has many treatment options, depending on its severity. They include medical therapy and surgical therapy, when patients have symptoms, or evidence of deterioration (such as a progressive increase in right heart size, reduction in systolic function, or the appearance of ventricular or atrial tachyarrhythmias). Electrical abnormalities may be associated with Ebstein's anomaly. In older children, radiofrequency ablation should be considered in such cases. In aortic valve insufficiency, afterload reduction may improve the left ventricular function and decrease regurgitant flow from the aorta. Surgical treatment should be considered when aortic valve insufficiency is severe, or if patients have symptoms and/or a reduction in their left ventricular function.

In patients with pulmonary regurgitation following TOF repair, although right ventricular volume load due to severe pulmonary regurgitation may be tolerated for years, there are some indications supporting pulmonary valve replacement before the onset of irreversible ventricular dysfunction. Geva published indications for pulmonary valve replacement in patients with moderate or severe PR with a regurgitation fraction of more than 25% on MRI, and two or more of the following criteria: right ventricular end-diastolic volume index of more than 160 ml/m2; right ventricular end-systolic volume index of more than 70 ml/m2; right ventricular ejection fraction of less than 45%; right ventricular outflow tract aneurysm; and the presence of symptoms [70]. In 2008, Frigiola *et al.* recommended that the presence of significant pulmonary regurgitation with regurgitation of more than 35% on MRI, with evidence of progression of right ventricular dilatation and dysfunction, and reduction in exercise capacity, are indications for pulmonary valve replacement [71]. Recommendations for timing and indications for pulmonary valve replacement indicated that early pulmonary valve replacement before the onset of symptoms of heart failure may reduce the risks of adverse clinical outcomes from chronic right ventricular volume load.

In young adults with right ventricular dysfunction after repair of TOF, beta-blocker therapy (such as bisoprolol) did not reduce circulating cytokines or improve ventricular function in asymptomatic or minimally symptomatic patients after six months of therapy [72].

Complex Congenital Heart Disease

Complex congenital heart diseases may affect both the systemic and pulmonary circulations, and can combine volume- and pressure-overload physiology. Palliative surgery, particularly the Fontan operation, is the palliative treatment for this group of patients. This operation has two stages: superior cavo-pulmonary anastomosis, followed by Fontan completion (in order to separate the systemic and pulmonary circulations, and only use the ventricle as the systemic ventricle). Moreover, Fontan completion at a younger age may reduce the operative mortality associated with this procedure to less than 5% (compared with 15-30% in the earlier decades), and survival at 20 years is presently around 85% [73].

Cardiomyopathy

Medical therapy, including inotropes and diuretics, should be used only to stabilize patients with cardiomyopathy associated with ALCAPA before surgery. Dobutamine or milrinone are beneficial to augment cardiac function. However, milrinone should be used cautiously, because it may cause systemic hypotension. The surgical for correction of ALCAPA involves the transfer of the anomalous left coronary artery to the aorta and usually results in improvement of the left ventricular function.

Besides standard heart failure therapy, determination of the aetiology of idiopathic DCM is essential to initiate treatment strategies. In adults with DCM, in whom a beta-blocker (such as carvedilol) is used, an increased stroke volume and stroke work index during exercise has been shown, along with a decreased heart rate and the LV chamber size. In addition, carvedilol has been shown to decrease pulmonary artery mean and wedge pressures, to decrease cardiac norepinephrine levels, and to increase peripheral vasodilation, particularly in cardiomyopathies. Clinical studies have also shown that carvedilol was beneficial for patients with symptomatic heart failure due to idiopathic DCM or ischaemic disease [74 - 76]. However, a double-blind, randomized trial between carvedilol and placebo in paediatric patients with mild to moderate congestive heart failure failed to demonstrate a benefit in terms of reduction of symptoms or mortality [77]. On the other hand, carvedilol may be effective in the prevention of the progression of diastolic dysfunction in patients with thalassaemia and dilated cardiomyopathy [78]. Carvedilol should only be introduced in stable patients, and the dose should be increased slowly. It must be stopped, if patients develop hypotension.

A worsening of the clinical conditions of heart failure patients may be precipitated by infective endocarditis, infections, anemia, electrolyte imbalance, arrhythmias, pulmonary embolism, drug interactions or toxicity. The treatment of these precipitating events results in a significant improvement. Nutrition is crucial in the management of paediatric heart failure, because of the increase in metabolic demands. Enhanced calorie content feeding, or nasogastric or gastrostomy feeding, may be necessary to maintain growth of the infant. Failure to thrive is an indication for increased medical management or, when the option is available, surgical repair of the congenital heart defects.

Mechanical Support

Many children with end-stage heart failure refractory to medical treatment may deteriorate and require short- or mid-term mechanical circulatory support (MCS), using veno-arterial extracorporeal membrane oxygenation (VA-ECMO) with a centrifugal pump, or long term MCS, using ventricular-assist devices (VADs) such as a Berlin Heart Excor or a Thoratec VAD. Both have been used temporarily as a supporting bridge to recovery or transplantation. The Excor was approved by the FDA in December 2011 and is available in graduated sizes to fit children from newborns to adolescents. However, the use of this device has a relatively high incidence of adverse side-effects, including a nearly 30% stroke rate [79].

Concerning the effect of LVAD on RV function is controversial. RV can occur in children with LVAD with an incidence of 42% in children. This could be due to increased RV overload together with leftward bowing of the the interventricular septum towards RV opposing RV contraction [80].

LVAD-related complications increase with the assistance duration. Hetzer *et al.* also noted that the optimal LV size and function occurs within approximately 90 days from LVAD implantation and then a gradual deterioration occurs during longer periods of support 21, 24. the RV dimensions increased over time after the pulsatile flow LVAD implantation. In addition, thanks to the reduction of the RV afterload due to the LVAD, the RVFAC improves in the short term follow up, but then it starts to decrease.

Heart Transplantation

Heart transplantation remains an acceptable treatment for children with end-stage heart failure. According to the registry of the International Society for Heart and Lung Transplantation, approximately 350-500 paediatric heart transplants are performed worldwide each year. Congenital heart defects, especially the hypoplastic left heart syndrome (HLHS), are the most common reason for infant heart transplantation, while cardiomyopathy is the commonest indication for heart transplantation in older children [81].

The goal of paediatric heart transplantation is to provide as much of a normal life span for these children as possible. The donor supply remains inadequate. Improved public and physician awareness of donor issues is the most important factor in increasing donor supply, because many potential donors are not identified.

CONCLUSION

Heart failure in children can be easily mistaken due to non-specific clinical presentation in infants and children, making the diagnosis difficult. Discovering the exact aetiology of heart failure in children may be challenging. However, many of the underlying causes are amenable to repair. As newer and better surgical and percutaneous treatment techniques and medications become available, resulting in improvement in the survival rates of children with heart failure as well as longer survival after transplantation, most children with heart failure should be able to reach adulthood and lead normal lives.

CONSENT FOR PUBLICATION

Not applicable.

CONFLICT OF INTEREST

The authors confirm that this chapter contents have no conflict of interest.

ACKNOWLEDGEMENTS

Declared none.

REFERENCES

[1]   Morrison LK, Harrison A, Krishnaswamy P, Kazanegra R, Clopton P, Maisel A. Utility of a rapid B-natriuretic peptide assay in differentiating congestive heart failure from lung disease in patients presenting with dyspnea. J Am Coll Cardiol 2002; 39(2): 202-9.
       [http://dx.doi.org/10.1016/S0735-1097(01)01744-2] [PMID: 11788208]

[2]   Dao Q, Krishnaswamy P, Kazanegra R, *et al.* Utility of B-type natriuretic peptide in the diagnosis of congestive heart failure in an urgent-care setting. J Am Coll Cardiol 2001; 37(2): 379-85.
       [http://dx.doi.org/10.1016/S0735-1097(00)01156-6] [PMID: 11216950]

[3]   Hirata Y, Matsumoto A, Aoyagi T, *et al.* Measurement of plasma brain natriuretic peptide level as a guide for cardiac overload. Cardiovasc Res 2001; 51(3): 585-91.
       [http://dx.doi.org/10.1016/S0008-6363(01)00320-0] [PMID: 11476749]

[4]   Wright GA, Struthers AD. Natriuretic peptides as a prognostic marker and therapeutic target in heart failure. Heart 2006; 92(2): 149-51.
       [http://dx.doi.org/10.1136/hrt.2003.018325] [PMID: 16216866]

[5]   Hsu DT, Pearson GD. Heart failure in children: part I: history, etiology, and pathophysiology. Circ Heart Fail 2009; 2(1): 63-70.
       [http://dx.doi.org/10.1161/CIRCHEARTFAILURE.108.820217] [PMID: 19808316]

[6]   Abu-Harb M, Hey E, Wren C. Death in infancy from unrecognised congenital heart disease. Arch Dis Child 1994; 71(1): 3-7.
[http://dx.doi.org/10.1136/adc.71.1.3] [PMID: 8067789]

[7]   Andrews RE, Fenton MJ, Ridout DA, Burch M. New-onset heart failure due to heart muscle disease in childhood: a prospective study in the United kingdom and Ireland. Circulation 2008; 117(1): 79-84.
[http://dx.doi.org/10.1161/CIRCULATIONAHA.106.671735] [PMID: 18086928]

[8]   Kantor PF, Mertens LL. Clinical practice: heart failure in children. Part I: clinical evaluation, diagnostic testing, and initial medical management. Eur J Pediatr 2010; 169(3): 269-79.
[http://dx.doi.org/10.1007/s00431-009-1024-y] [PMID: 19707788]

[9]   Erickson LC. Medical issues for the cardiac patient. Critical Care of Infants and Children 1996; pp. 259-62.

[10]   Ross RD, Daniels SR, Schwartz DC, Hannon DW, Shukla R, Kaplan S. Plasma norepinephrine levels in infants and children with congestive heart failure. Am J Cardiol 1987; 59(8): 911-4.
[http://dx.doi.org/10.1016/0002-9149(87)91118-0] [PMID: 3825955]

[11]   Johnstone DE, Abdulla A, Arnold JM, et al. Diagnosis and management of heart failure. Can J Cardiol 1994; 10(6): 613-631, 635-654.
[PMID: 8044722]

[12]   The Criteria Committee of the New York Heart Association Nomenclature and criteria for diagnosis of diseases of the heart and blood vessels. Boston: Little Brown 1964.

[13]   Yancy CW, Jessup M, Bozkurt B, et al. 2013 ACCF/AHA guideline for the management of heart failure: executive summary: a report of the American College of Cardiology Foundation/American Heart Association Task Force on practice guidelines. Circulation 2013; 128(16): 1810-52.
[http://dx.doi.org/10.1161/CIR.0b013e31829e8807] [PMID: 23741057]

[14]   Pasquali SK, Hall M, Slonim AD, et al. Off-label use of cardiovascular medications in children hospitalized with congenital and acquired heart disease. Circ Cardiovasc Qual Outcomes 2008; 1(2): 74-83.
[http://dx.doi.org/10.1161/CIRCOUTCOMES.108.787176] [PMID: 20031793]

[15]   Tissières P, Aggoun Y, Da Cruz E, et al. Comparison of classifications for heart failure in children undergoing valvular surgery. J Pediatr 2006; 149(2): 210-5.
[http://dx.doi.org/10.1016/j.jpeds.2006.04.006] [PMID: 16887436]

[16]   Keane MG, Wiegers SE, Plappert T, Pochettino A, Bavaria JE, Sutton MG. Bicuspid aortic valves are associated with aortic dilatation out of proportion to coexistent valvular lesions. Circulation 2000; 102(19) (Suppl. 3): III35-9.
[http://dx.doi.org/10.1161/01.CIR.102.suppl_3.III-35] [PMID: 11082359]

[17]   Khairy P, Poirier N, Mercier LA. Univentricular heart. Circulation 2007; 115(6): 800-12.
[http://dx.doi.org/10.1161/CIRCULATIONAHA.105.592378] [PMID: 17296869]

[18]   McRae ME. Long-term issues after the Fontan procedure. AACN Adv Crit Care 2013; 24(3): 264-82.
[http://dx.doi.org/10.1097/NCI.0b013e31829744c7] [PMID: 23880749]

[19]   Dahle G, Fiane AE, Lindberg HL. ALCAPA, a possible reason for mitral insufficiency and heart failure in young patients. Scand Cardiovasc J 2007; 41(1): 51-8.
[http://dx.doi.org/10.1080/14017430601050348] [PMID: 17365978]

[20]   Elshazly MB, Pettersson G, Thamilarasan M. High-output heart failure secondary to anomalous left coronary artery from pulmonary in an adult. J Am Coll Cardiol 2015; 65: 10S.
[http://dx.doi.org/10.1016/S0735-1097(15)60586-1]

[21]   Kristensen T, Kofoed KF, Helqvist S, Helvind M, Søndergaard L. Anomalous origin of the left coronary artery from the pulmonary artery (ALCAPA) presenting with ventricular fibrillation in an adult: a case report. J Cardiothorac Surg 2008; 3: 33.

[http://dx.doi.org/10.1186/1749-8090-3-33] [PMID: 18503713]

[22] Lipshultz SE, Sleeper LA, Towbin JA, *et al.* The incidence of pediatric cardiomyopathy in two regions of the United States. N Engl J Med 2003; 348(17): 1647-55.
[http://dx.doi.org/10.1056/NEJMoa021715] [PMID: 12711739]

[23] Nugent AW, Daubeney PE, Chondros P, *et al.* The epidemiology of childhood cardiomyopathy in Australia. N Engl J Med 2003; 348(17): 1639-46.
[http://dx.doi.org/10.1056/NEJMoa021737] [PMID: 12711738]

[24] Strauss A, Lock JE. Pediatric cardiomyopathy--a long way to go. N Engl J Med 2003; 348(17): 1703-5.
[http://dx.doi.org/10.1056/NEJMe030027] [PMID: 12711746]

[25] Madriago E, Silberbach M. Heart failure in infants and children. Pediatr Rev 2010; 31(1): 4-12.
[http://dx.doi.org/10.1542/pir.31-1-4] [PMID: 20048034]

[26] Sen-Chowdhry S, McKenna WJ. Sudden Cardiac Death. Sudden Death From Genetic and Acquired Cardiomyopathies Circulation 2012; 125: 1563-76.
[PMID: 22451606]

[27] Lipshultz SE, Cochran TR, Briston DA, *et al.* Pediatric cardiomyopathies: causes, epidemiology, clinical course, preventive strategies and therapies. Future Cardiol 2013; 9(6): 817-48.
[http://dx.doi.org/10.2217/fca.13.66] [PMID: 24180540]

[28] Kantor PF, Lougheed J, Dancea A, *et al.* Presentation, diagnosis, and medical management of heart failure in children: Canadian Cardiovascular Society guidelines. Can J Cardiol 2013; 29(12): 1535-52.
[http://dx.doi.org/10.1016/j.cjca.2013.08.008] [PMID: 24267800]

[29] Towbin JA, Lowe AM, Colan SD, *et al.* Incidence, causes, and outcomes of dilated cardiomyopathy in children. JAMA 2006; 296(15): 1867-76.
[http://dx.doi.org/10.1001/jama.296.15.1867] [PMID: 17047217]

[30] Williams RV, Ritter S, Tani LY, Pagoto LT, Minich LL. Quantitative assessment of ventricular function in children with single ventricles using the Doppler myocardial performance index. Am J Cardiol 2000; 86(10): 1106-10.
[http://dx.doi.org/10.1016/S0002-9149(00)01168-1] [PMID: 11074208]

[31] Hsu DT, Pearson GD. Heart failure in children: part II: diagnosis, treatment, and future directions. Circ Heart Fail 2009; 2(5): 490-8.
[http://dx.doi.org/10.1161/CIRCHEARTFAILURE.109.856229] [PMID: 19808380]

[32] Taylor AM. Cardiac imaging: MR or CT? Which to use when. Pediatr Radiol 2008; 38 (Suppl. 3): S433-8.
[http://dx.doi.org/10.1007/s00247-008-0843-8] [PMID: 18470452]

[33] Kilner PJ, Geva T, Kaemmerer H, Trindade PT, Schwitter J, Webb GD. Recommendations for cardiovascular magnetic resonance in adults with congenital heart disease from the respective working groups of the European Society of Cardiology. Eur Heart J 2010; 31(7): 794-805.
[http://dx.doi.org/10.1093/eurheartj/ehp586] [PMID: 20067914]

[34] Pennell DJ, Sechtem UP, Higgins CB, *et al.* Clinical indications for cardiovascular magnetic resonance (CMR): Consensus Panel report. Eur Heart J 2004; 25(21): 1940-65.
[http://dx.doi.org/10.1016/j.ehj.2004.06.040] [PMID: 15522474]

[35] Powell AJ, Geva T. Blood flow measurement by magnetic resonance imaging in congenital heart disease. Pediatr Cardiol 2000; 21(1): 47-58.
[http://dx.doi.org/10.1007/s002469910007] [PMID: 10672614]

[36] Beerbaum P, Körperich H, Barth P, Esdorn H, Gieseke J, Meyer H. Noninvasive quantification of left-to-right shunt in pediatric patients: phase-contrast cine magnetic resonance imaging compared with invasive oximetry. Circulation 2001; 103(20): 2476-82.
[http://dx.doi.org/10.1161/01.CIR.103.20.2476] [PMID: 11369688]

[37]   Cheitlin MD, Armstrong WF, Aurigemma GP, *et al.* ACC/AHA/ASE 2003 guideline update for the clinical application of echocardiography: summary article: a report of the American College of Cardiology/American Heart Association task force on practice guidelines (ACC/AHA/ASE committee to update the 1997 guidelines for the clinical application of echocardiography). J Am Coll Cardiol 2003; 42(5): 954-70.
[http://dx.doi.org/10.1016/S0735-1097(03)01065-9] [PMID: 12957449]

[38]   Gulati A, Jabbour A, Ismail TF, *et al.* Association of fibrosis with mortality and sudden cardiac death in patients with nonischemic dilated cardiomyopathy. JAMA 2013; 309(9): 896-908.
[http://dx.doi.org/10.1001/jama.2013.1363] [PMID: 23462786]

[39]   Higgins CB, Byrd BF III, Farmer DW, Osaki L, Silverman NH, Cheitlin MD. Magnetic resonance imaging in patients with congenital heart disease. Circulation 1984; 70(5): 851-60.
[http://dx.doi.org/10.1161/01.CIR.70.5.851] [PMID: 6488498]

[40]   Riesenkampff E, Messroghli D, Redington A, *et al.* Translating novel imaging technologies into clinical applications: Myocardial T1 mapping in pediatric and congenital heart disease. Circ Cardiovasc Imaging 2015; 8: 1-130.
[http://dx.doi.org/10.1161/CIRCIMAGING.114.002504]

[41]   Ntsinjana HN, Hughes ML, Taylor AM. The role of cardiovascular magnetic resonance in pediatric congenital heart disease. J Cardiovasc Magn Reson 2011; 13: 51-71.
[http://dx.doi.org/10.1186/1532-429X-13-51] [PMID: 21936913]

[42]   Auerbach SR, Richmond ME, Lamour JM, *et al.* BNP levels predict outcome in pediatric heart failure patients: post hoc analysis of the Pediatric Carvedilol Trial. Circ Heart Fail 2010; 3(5): 606-11.
[http://dx.doi.org/10.1161/CIRCHEARTFAILURE.109.906875] [PMID: 20573993]

[43]   Tang WH, Francis GS, Morrow DA, *et al.* National Academy of Clinical Biochemistry Laboratory Medicine practice guidelines: Clinical utilization of cardiac biomarker testing in heart failure. Circulation 2007; 116(5): e99-e109.
[PMID: 17630410]

[44]   Price JF, Thomas AK, Grenier M, *et al.* B-type natriuretic peptide predicts adverse cardiovascular events in pediatric outpatients with chronic left ventricular systolic dysfunction. Circulation 2006; 114(10): 1063-9.
[http://dx.doi.org/10.1161/CIRCULATIONAHA.105.608869] [PMID: 16940194]

[45]   Hershberger RE, Lindenfeld J, Mestroni L, Seidman CE, Taylor MR, Towbin JA. Genetic evaluation of cardiomyopathy--a Heart Failure Society of America practice guideline. J Card Fail 2009; 15(2): 83-97.
[http://dx.doi.org/10.1016/j.cardfail.2009.01.006] [PMID: 19254666]

[46]   Høst A, Halken S, Kamper J, Lillquist K. Prostaglandin E1 treatment in ductus dependent congenital cardiac malformation. A review of the treatment of 34 neonates. Dan Med Bull 1988; 35(1): 81-4.
[PMID: 3342648]

[47]   Kramer HH, Sommer M, Rammos S, Krogmann O. Evaluation of low dose prostaglandin E1 treatment for ductus dependent congenital heart disease. Eur J Pediatr 1995; 154(9): 700-7.
[http://dx.doi.org/10.1007/BF02276712] [PMID: 8582419]

[48]   Robertson CM, Tyebkhan JM, Peliowski A, Etches PC, Cheung PY. Ototoxic drugs and sensorineural hearing loss following severe neonatal respiratory failure. Acta Paediatr 2006; 95(2): 214-23.
[http://dx.doi.org/10.1080/08035250500294098] [PMID: 16449030]

[49]   Berman W Jr, Yabek SM, Dillon T, Niland C, Corlew S, Christensen D. Effects of digoxin in infants with congested circulatory state due to a ventricular septal defect. N Engl J Med 1983; 308(7): 363-6.
[http://dx.doi.org/10.1056/NEJM198302173080704] [PMID: 6296675]

[50]   Seguchi M, Nakazawa M, Momma K. Further evidence suggesting a limited role of digitalis in infants with a congested circulatory state due to a ventricular septal defect. Am J Cardiol 1999; 83: 1408-11.

[http://dx.doi.org/10.1016/S0002-9149(99)00109-5] [PMID: 10235104]

[51]   Berg RA, Donnerstein RL, Padbury JF. Dobutamine infusions in stable, critically ill children: pharmacokinetics and hemodynamic actions. Crit Care Med 1993; 21(5): 678-86.
[http://dx.doi.org/10.1097/00003246-199305000-00010] [PMID: 8482088]

[52]   Martinez AM, Padbury JF, Thio S. Dobutamine pharmacokinetics and cardiovascular responses in critically ill neonates. Pediatrics 1992; 89(1): 47-51.
[PMID: 1728020]

[53]   Leier CV, Webel J, Bush CA. The cardiovascular effects of the continuous infusion of dobutamine in patients with severe cardiac failure. Circulation 1977; 56(3): 468-72.
[http://dx.doi.org/10.1161/01.CIR.56.3.468] [PMID: 884803]

[54]   Hoffman TM, Wernovsky G, Atz AM, *et al.* Efficacy and safety of milrinone in preventing low cardiac output syndrome in infants and children after corrective surgery for congenital heart disease. Circulation 2003; 107(7): 996-1002.
[http://dx.doi.org/10.1161/01.CIR.0000051365.81920.28] [PMID: 12600913]

[55]   Shaddy RE, Teitel DF, Brett C. Short-term hemodynamic effects of captopril in infants with congestive heart failure. Am J Dis Child 1988; 142(1): 100-5.
[PMID: 3277384]

[56]   Scammell AM, Arnold R, Wilkinson JL. Captopril in treatment of infant heart failure: a preliminary report. Int J Cardiol 1987; 16(3): 295-301.
[http://dx.doi.org/10.1016/0167-5273(87)90153-7] [PMID: 3308715]

[57]   Engle MA, Lewy JE, Lewy PR, Metcoff J. The use of furosemide in the treatment of edema in infants and children. Pediatrics 1978; 62(5): 811-8.
[PMID: 724325]

[58]   Pitt B, Zannad F, Remme WJ, *et al.* The effect of spironolactone on morbidity and mortality in patients with severe heart failure. N Engl J Med 1999; 341(10): 709-17.
[http://dx.doi.org/10.1056/NEJM199909023411001] [PMID: 10471456]

[59]   Frenneaux M, Stewart RA, Newman CM, Hallidie-Smith KA. Enalapril for severe heart failure in infancy. Arch Dis Child 1989; 64(2): 219-23.
[http://dx.doi.org/10.1136/adc.64.2.219] [PMID: 2539059]

[60]   Sluysmans T, Styns-Cailteux M, Tremouroux-Wattiez M, *et al.* Intravenous enalaprilat and oral enalapril in congestive heart failure secondary to ventricular septal defect in infancy. Am J Cardiol 1992; 70(9): 959-62.
[http://dx.doi.org/10.1016/0002-9149(92)90749-O] [PMID: 1326889]

[61]   Momma K. ACE inhibitors in pediatric patients with heart failure. Paediatr Drugs 2006; 8(1): 55-69.
[http://dx.doi.org/10.2165/00148581-200608010-00005] [PMID: 16494512]

[62]   Margossian R. Contemporary management of pediatric heart failure. Expert Rev Cardiovasc Ther 2008; 6(2): 187-97.
[http://dx.doi.org/10.1586/14779072.6.2.187] [PMID: 18248273]

[63]   Wiyono SA, Witsenburg M, de Jaegere PP, Roos-Hesselink JW. Patent ductus arteriosus in adults: Case report and review illustrating the spectrum of the disease. Neth Heart J 2008; 16(7-8): 255-9.
[http://dx.doi.org/10.1007/BF03086157] [PMID: 18711613]

[64]   Hofstetter R, Zeike B, Messmer BJ, von Bernuth G. Echocardiographic evaluation of systolic left-ventricular function in infants with critical aortic stenosis before and after aortic valvotomy. Thorac Cardiovasc Surg 1990; 38(4): 236-40.
[http://dx.doi.org/10.1055/s-2007-1014024] [PMID: 2237884]

[65]   Mosca RS, Iannettoni MD, Schwartz SM, *et al.* Critical aortic stenosis in the neonate. A comparison of balloon valvuloplasty and transventricular dilation. J Thorac Cardiovasc Surg 1995; 109(1): 147-54.
[http://dx.doi.org/10.1016/S0022-5223(95)70430-2] [PMID: 7815791]

[66] Feltes TF, Bacha E, Beekman RH III, *et al.* Indications for cardiac catheterization and intervention in pediatric cardiac disease: a scientific statement from the American Heart Association. Circulation 2011; 123(22): 2607-52.
[http://dx.doi.org/10.1161/CIR.0b013e31821b1f10] [PMID: 21536996]

[67] Rocchini AP, Beekman RH, Ben Shachar G, Benson L, Schwartz D, Kan JS. Balloon aortic valvuloplasty: results of the valvuloplasty and angioplasty of congenital anomalies registry. Am J Cardiol 1990; 65(11): 784-9.
[http://dx.doi.org/10.1016/0002-9149(90)91388-M] [PMID: 2316461]

[68] Keane JF, Driscoll DJ, Gersony WM, *et al.* Second natural history study of congenital heart defects. Results of treatment of patients with aortic valvar stenosis. Circulation 1993; 87(2) (Suppl.): I16-27.
[PMID: 8425319]

[69] Justo RN, McCrindle BW, Benson LN, Williams WG, Freedom RM, Smallhorn JF. Aortic valve regurgitation after surgical *versus* percutaneous balloon valvotomy for congenital aortic valve stenosis. Am J Cardiol 1996; 77(15): 1332-8.
[http://dx.doi.org/10.1016/S0002-9149(96)00201-9] [PMID: 8677875]

[70] Geva T. Indications and timing of pulmonary valve replacement after tetralogy of Fallot repair. Semin Thorac Cardiovasc Surg Pediatr Card Surg Annu 2006; •••: 11-22.
[http://dx.doi.org/10.1053/j.pcsu.2006.02.009] [PMID: 16638542]

[71] Frigiola A, Tsang V, Nordmeyer J, *et al.* Current approaches to pulmonary regurgitation. Eur J Cardiothorac Surg 2008; 34(3): 576-80.
[http://dx.doi.org/10.1016/j.ejcts.2008.04.046] [PMID: 18539471]

[72] Norozi K, Buchhorn R, Wessel A, *et al.* Beta-blockade does not alter plasma cytokine concentrations and ventricular function in young adults with right ventricular dysfunction secondary to operated congenital heart disease. Circ J 2008; 72(5): 747-52.
[http://dx.doi.org/10.1253/circj.72.747] [PMID: 18441454]

[73] d'Udekem Y, Iyengar AJ, Cochrane AD, *et al.* The Fontan procedure: contemporary techniques have improved long-term outcomes. Circulation 2007; 116(11) (Suppl.): I157-64.
[http://dx.doi.org/10.1161/CIRCULATIONAHA.106.676445] [PMID: 17846297]

[74] Packer M, Colucci WS, Sackner-Bernstein JD, *et al.* Double-blind, placebo-controlled study of the effects of carvedilol in patients with moderate to severe heart failure. The PRECISE Trial. Prospective Randomized Evaluation of Carvedilol on Symptoms and Exercise. Circulation 1996; 94(11): 2793-9.
[http://dx.doi.org/10.1161/01.CIR.94.11.2793] [PMID: 8941104]

[75] Metra M, Nardi M, Giubbini R, Dei Cas L. Effects of short- and long-term carvedilol administration on rest and exercise hemodynamic variables, exercise capacity and clinical conditions in patients with idiopathic dilated cardiomyopathy. J Am Coll Cardiol 1994; 24(7): 1678-87.
[http://dx.doi.org/10.1016/0735-1097(94)90174-0] [PMID: 7963115]

[76] Chizzola PR, Freitas HF, Caldas MA, *et al.* Effects of carvedilol in heart failure due to dilated cardiomyopathy. Results of a double-blind randomized placebo-controlled study (CARIBE study). Arq Bras Cardiol 2000; 74(3): 233-42.
[http://dx.doi.org/10.1590/S0066-782X2000000300005] [PMID: 10951826]

[77] Shaddy RE, Boucek MM, Hsu DT, *et al.* Carvedilol for children and adolescents with heart failure: a randomized controlled trial. JAMA 2007; 298(10): 1171-9.
[http://dx.doi.org/10.1001/jama.298.10.1171] [PMID: 17848651]

[78] Ajami GH, Amoozgar H, Borzouee M, *et al.* Efficacy of carvedilol in patients with dilated cardiomyopathy due to beta-thalassemia major; a double-blind randomized controlled trial. Iran J Pediatr 2010; 20(3): 277-83.
[PMID: 23056717]

[79] Fraser CD Jr, Jaquiss RD, Rosenthal DN, *et al.* Prospective trial of a pediatric ventricular assist device.

N Engl J Med 2012; 367(6): 532-41.
[http://dx.doi.org/10.1056/NEJMoa1014164] [PMID: 22873533]

[80]   Di Molfetta A, Iacobelli R, Filippelli S, *et al.* Evolution of Biventricular Loading Condition in Pediatric LVAD Patient: A Prospective and Observational Study. Artif Organs 2018; 42(4): 386-93.
[http://dx.doi.org/10.1111/aor.13050] [PMID: 29230826]

[81]   Dipchand AI, Edwards LB, Kucheryavaya AY, *et al.* The registry of the International Society for Heart and Lung Transplantation: seventeenth official pediatric heart transplantation report--2014; focus theme: retransplantation. J Heart Lung Transplant 2014; 33(10): 985-95.
[http://dx.doi.org/10.1016/j.healun.2014.08.002] [PMID: 25242123]

CHAPTER 2

Heart Failure in Pediatric Patients with Congenital Heart Disease

Anas Taqatqa[1], Mohammad El Tahlawi[2], Kasey J. Chaszczewski[1] and Sawsan Awad[1,*]

[1] *Rush University Medical Center, Chicago, USA*

[2] *Zagazig University, Zagazig, Egypt*

Abstract: Heart failure may occur in structurally normal heart or in congenitally diseased heart. Some congenital heart diseases may predispose to heart failure, in different mechanisms and different pictures, as Fallot tetralogy, single ventricle, muscular dystrophy associated cardiomyopathy and left ventricular non compaction. The etiology of heart failure in those patients may be due to volume overload, pressure overload or valve insufficiency. The medical treatment for such patients includes diuretics, B blockers, ACE inhibitors, digoxin and anticoagulations.

Keywords: Atrial Septal Defect, Biomarkers, Cardiomyopathy, Congenital Heart Disease, Echocardiography, Fontan, Heart Failure, Single Ventricle, Tetralogy of Fallot.

INTRODUCTION

Heart failure (HF) is a progressive clinical syndrome characterized by elevated filling pressure and/or obstruction to blood ejection leading to neurohormonal system activation and molecular derangements. Diagnosis of HF depends on identification of a constellation of symptoms, signs and multiple non-invasive and invasive diagnostic studies as echocardiography, cardiac MRI, exercise testing, biomarkers and cardiac catheterization [1, 2]. Extensive effort should be made to identify the etiology of HF for prognostic classification and creation of appropriate management plan.

Variable causes of HF in children have been identified. Classification and sub-classification of HF etiologies allow better understanding of the pathophysiology of HF and permit tailoring of treatment plan.

---

* **Corresponding author Sawsan Awad:** Rush University Medical Center Chicago, IL 60612 ; Tel: 3129427496; Fax: 3129426801; E-mail: sawsan_m_awad@rush.edu

Mohammad El Tahlawi (Ed.)
All rights reserved-© 2020 Bentham Science Publishers

Two major etiologic categories have been identified; HF in structurally normal heart (SNH) and HF in Congenital Heart Disease (CHD) [3]. Table **1** summarizes the etiologic causes of HF in children.

Table 1. Causes of heart failure in children.

Congenital:
Volume overload
Shunts:
Ventricular septal defect
Patent ductus arteriosus
Atrioventricular septal defect
Truncus arteriosus
Valve Insufficiency:
Atrioventricular valve insufficiency (*e.g.* atrioventricular canal)
Aortic regurgitation in bicuspid aortic valve
Pulmonary regurgitation after repair of tetralogy of Fallot
Truncal valve regurgitation
Pressure overload
Severe aortic stenosis
Coarctation of the aorta
Severe pulmonary stenosis
Complex congenital heart disease
Single ventricle
Hypoplastic left heart syndrome
Unbalanced atrioventricular septal defect
Systemic right ventricle
Congenitally corrected transposition of the great artery
Post Mustard/Senning procedures
Structurally normal heart
Primary cardiomyopathy
Dilated
Hypertrophic
Restrictive
Secondary cardiomyopathy
Infectious (myocarditis, endocarditis)
Ischemia (Kawasaki disease, anomalous left coronary artery from the pulmonary artery)
Chronic arrhythmias
Toxins (anthracyclines)
Metabolic
Infectious

HF in SNH Includes

1. Patients with primary cardiomyopathies as dilated, hypertrophic and restrictive cardiomyopathies

2. Patients with HF secondary to primary disease as ischemic cardiomyopathy,

infiltrative cardiomyopathy and cardiomyopathy secondary to chronic arrhythmia (arrhythmogenic).

HF in CHD Includes

1. HF secondary to volume overload as in left to right shunt lesions (ventricular septal defect (VSD), and patent ductus arteriosus (PDA) and in cardiac valve regurgitation lesions.
2. HF secondary to pressure overload as in patients with left or right sided obstructive lesions
3. HF in patients with complex CHD as patients with single ventricle physiology and systemic right ventricle.

In this chapter, HF in selected lesions will be discussed. Medical and surgical management of HF will be reviewed at the end of this chapter.

Tetralogy of Fallot

Tetralogy of Fallot (TOF) is the most common cyanotic congenital heart disease. It has four cardinal features: anterior malalignment of VSD, pulmonary valve and right ventricle (RV) outflow narrowing, over-riding of the aorta, and RV hypertrophy. The goals of complete surgical repair are VSD patch closure and relief of the RV outflow/pulmonary valve obstruction. This may entail sacrificing the pulmonary valve with subsequent pulmonary valve regurgitation.

HF in patients with uncorrected TOF is a rare occurrence due to standard early surgical repair in infancy in United States of America and most of the European countries. Older patients with unrepaired TOF present with severe chronic hypoxia and myocardial ischemia secondary to thrombotic occlusion of the coronary arteries leading to cardiomyopathy and subsequently HF [4, 5].

On the other hand, patients with repaired TOF may present with HF due to several contributing factors namely chronic pulmonary regurgitation (PR), tricuspid regurgitation (TR), residual RV outflow obstruction, ventricular fibrosis and electrophysiological abnormalities.

Progressive PR has long-term deleterious effect on the RV function. Chronic volume overload initially results in compensatory RV dilatation and hypertrophy. Patients are frequently asymptomatic years following the initial surgical repair, though cardiopulmonary exercise testing showed reduced exercise capacity earlier than it was previously thought [6]. TR, if present, aggravates the RV dilation, which leads to more regurgitation and eventually more dilation [7]. RV dysfunction may develop over time, which leads to irreversible myocardial damage if not addressed early in the process. Additionally, ventricular fibrosis plays an important role in myocardial dysfunction and the development of arrhythmia and HF. Ventricular fibrosis may arise in the area of previous myocardial resection in the RV outflow, in relation to the area of patch suture or intraoperative vent insertion. Older age at repair was found to increase the extent of myocardial fibrosis [8].

Some patients develop impairment of diastolic function, specifically the late diastolic filling. This phenomenon was initially diagnosed by echocardiography using pulse wave Doppler measurement which shows ante-grade pulmonary arterial flow in late diastole (Fig. **1**) [9]. More recently, tissue Doppler and strain rate (Figs. **2** and **3**) evaluation of these patients provide early and accurate noninvasive diagnosis of RV diastolic impairment [10]. Patients with diastolic dysfunction usually develop postoperative low cardiac output syndrome due to impaired RV filling. This syndrome is more pronounced in the presence of significant PR [11]. Discordant results have been reported on the long-term effect of restrictive RV physiology on patients' RV volume and wellbeing. One study showed lower cardiothoracic ratio by chest radiography and better exercise tolerance which points to the beneficial effect of RV restrictive physiology [12]. Another report showed no difference in measured RV volume by cardiac MRI and reduced exercise capacity compared to patients without RV restrictive physiology. The study evaluated children hence there is potentially short time for the RV to dilate in those patients without restrictive RV [13].

Interaction between RV and left ventricle (LV) is fundamental to normal cardiac function. RV dilation and paradoxical wall motion of the ventricular septum impair LV filling pressure and cause poor ventricular synchrony. (Video clips 1-4). Several studies showed an association between RV dysfunction and depressed LV ejection fraction (EF) [14, 15]. Additionally, the presence of moderate or severe LV systolic dysfunction in TOF patients with RV dilation increased the incidence of sudden cardiac death [16]. LV EF improved significantly following pulmonary valve replacement in addition to its well-known beneficial effect on RV function and size [17].

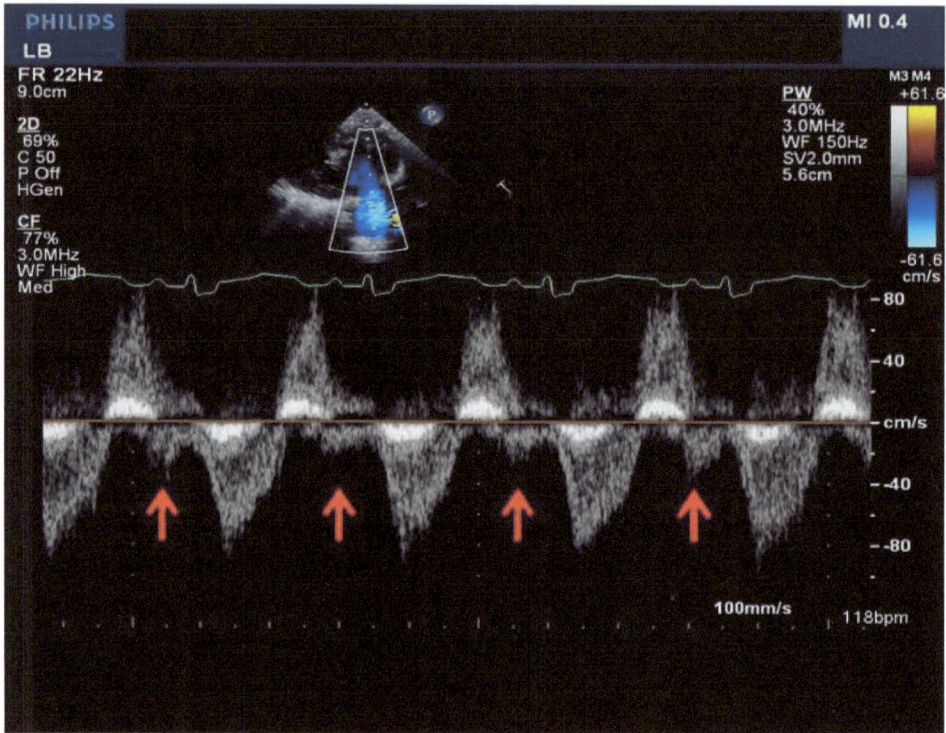

Fig. (1). Pulsed wave Doppler performed across the pulmonary valve of in a patient with tetralogy of Fallot, significant pulmonary valve regurgitation and RV diastolic dysfunction. The tracing shows ante-grade pulmonary arterial flow in late diastole (Red arrows).

Physical assessment, echocardiography, ECG and cardiopulmonary exercise testing are recommended for routine monitoring of patients with repaired TOF. Cardiac MRI has been used increasingly to quantify the RV and LV volumes and function. Patients with absolute contraindication(s) to MRI can receive cardiac computed tomography evaluation with as accurate quantification of the RV volume and ejection fraction as in MRI (Figs. **4** and **5**) [18]. A recent report showed that Ramipril (an ACE inhibitor) has improved biventricular function in repaired TOF patients. Large sample size and longer term follow up are required to evaluate the overall clinical outcome [19]. B-blockers failed to show significant impact on the clinical status and RV function [20]. Classical therapeutic options include surgical or interventional pulmonary valve replacement and elimination of distal pulmonary artery obstructive lesions if present.

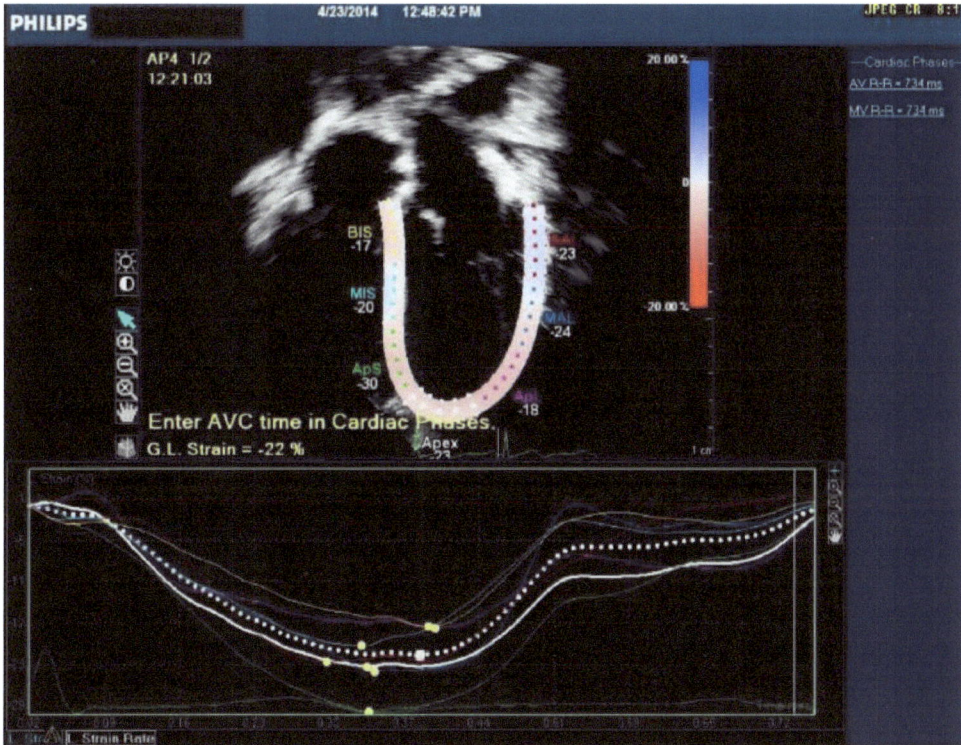

Fig. (2). Speckle tracking echocardiography to evaluate the longitudinal strain in an apical 4-chamber view of a patient with normal myocardial function. The color points or speckles track the left ventricular borders. The global longitudinal strain (G.L. strain) value is listed in addition to the segmental longitudinal strain values. Values more than -17 are considered to be normal.

Single Ventricle

In contrary to TOF, single ventricle (SV) is rare. Its incidence is about 1% of patients with congenital heart disease. SV includes lesions where both right and left atria are connected to one ventricle. That ventricle can be a single LV, a single RV or a common ventricle with mixed morphology. Other congenital heart lesions as hypoplastic left heart syndrome (HLHS) and tricuspid atresia (TA) are not considered to be true lesions although they have the same pathophysiology as SV. HLHS and TA patients are categorized as patients with SV physiology or functional SV.

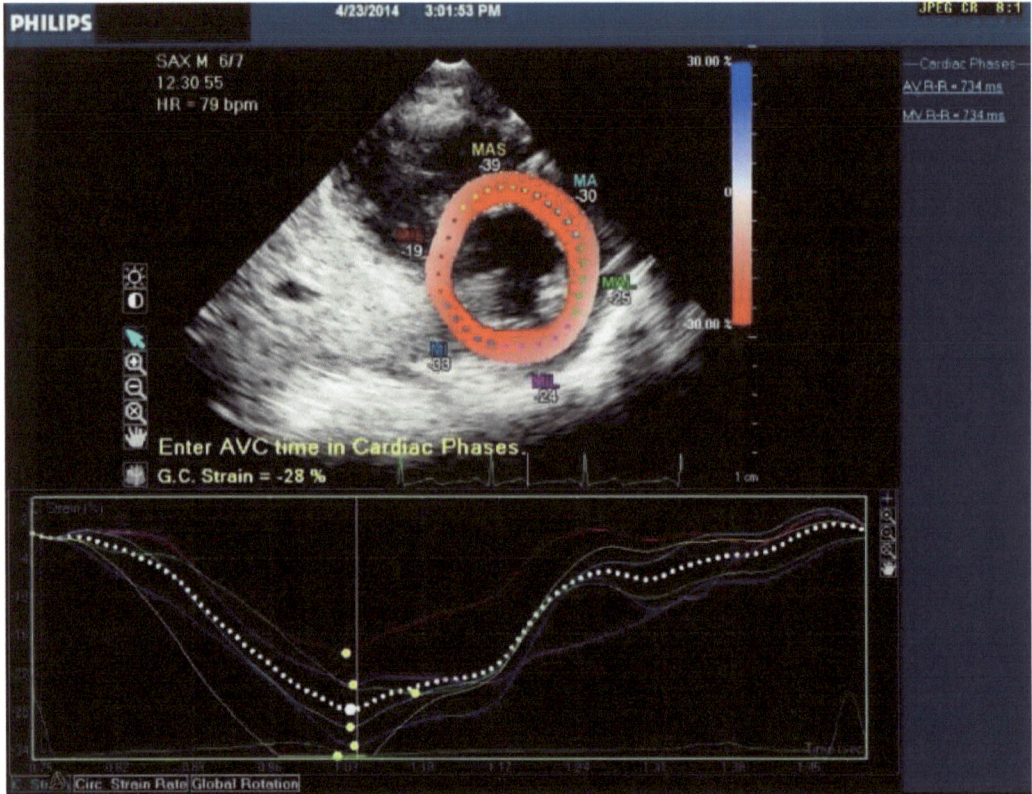

Fig. (3). Speckle tracking echocardiography to evaluate the circumferential strain in parasternal short axis view, mid-left ventricular portion. The global circumferential strain (G.C. strain) value is listed in addition to the segmental circumferential strain values. Values more than -17 are considered to be normal.

In the true SV, both atria open into a single ventricle *via* either a common atrioventricular valve (common inlet) or two atrioventricular valves (double inlet). The most common type of SV lesions is double inlet left ventricle. In this lesion, the single ventricle has LV morphology while the atretic chamber is of RV morphology and is located into the left and anterior of the dominant LV (L-looping). The diminutive RV usually gives rise to the aorta. The two ventricles are usually connected through a ventricular septal defect type of lesion, which is called bulboventricular foramen.

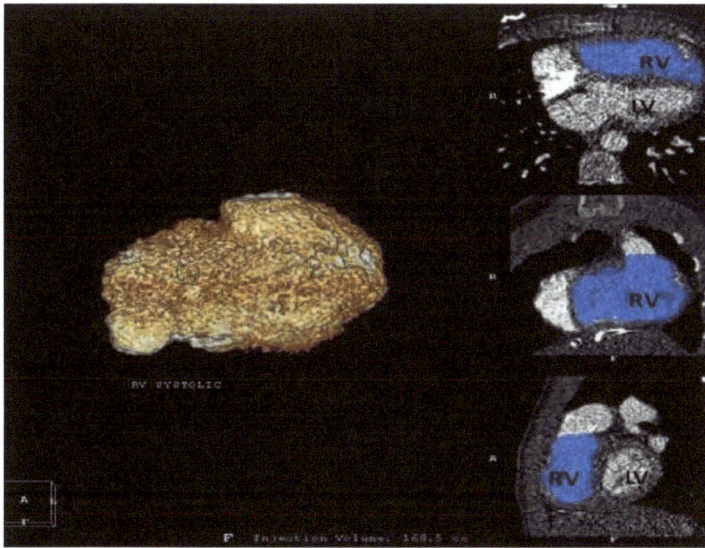

Fig. (4). CT angiogram of a 17 year old male patient with tetralogy of Fallot and a pacemaker hence cardiac MRI was contraindicated. The right ventricular systolic volume is evaluated in 3 different CT cuts (longitudinal-top right, oblique-mid right, and short axis-lower right). The final right ventricular systolic volume is given in the left middle reconstructed volume tracing.

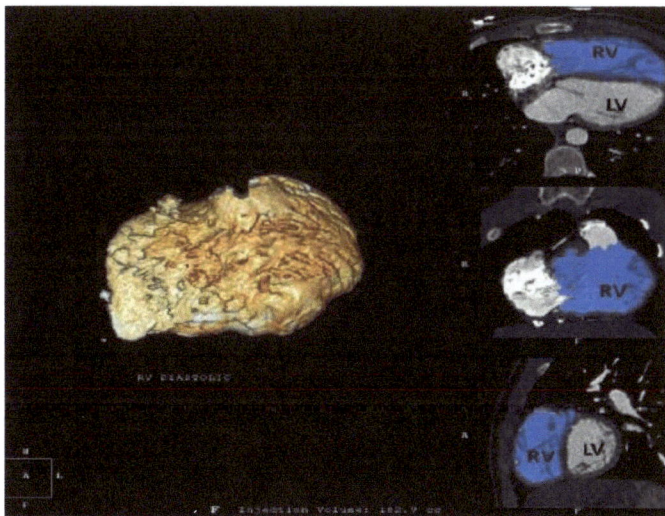

Fig. (5). CT angiogram of the same patient in Fig. (4). The right ventricular diastolic volume is evaluated in 3 different CT cuts (longitudinal-top right, oblique-mid right, and short axis-lower right). The final right ventricular diastolic volume is given in the left middle reconstructed volume tracing.

The amount of pulmonary blood flow determines the degree of cyanosis. The pulmonary blood flow in these patients depends on the degree of pulmonary stenosis and the pulmonary vascular resistance. Three variable presentations may be encountered. The first presentation is in patients with mild to moderate pulmonary stenosis who have just enough pulmonary blood flow. No initial intervention is needed in this group of patients and they are referred to as naturally banded. The second presentation is in patients with pulmonary atresia and no forward pulmonary blood flow. This group of patients will have significant cyanosis and require a source of pulmonary blood supply, initially in the form of maintaining patency of the arterial duct. Finally is the presentation in patients with no pulmonary stenosis. These patients subsequently develop symptoms and signs of increased pulmonary blood flow once the pulmonary vascular resistance normalizes. These patients will require banding of the main pulmonary artery to mechanically restrict the pulmonary blood flow.

As explained above, the three variable initial presentations dictate different initial surgical treatment plans (stage I surgery). Stage I surgery usually takes place in the first 2-3 weeks of age. All patients subsequently undergo superior cavopulmonary anastomosis (Glenn procedure) at 3-6 months of age followed by total cavopulmonary anastomosis (Fontan procedure) at 2-3 years of age [21] [22].

In extreme forms of HLHS, mitral and aortic valve atresia together with hypoplastic aortic arch and severe hypoplasia of LV are present. Systemic cardiac output is supplied by the right ventricle through the patent ductus arteriosus (PDA). Infants with HLHS usually do well in utero. In the neonatal period, maintaining the patency of the ductus arteriosus is crucial for survival. The systemic circulation relies exclusively on flow through the PDA from the right ventricle. This will feed both the descending and ascending aorta.

Blood ejected from the right ventricle supplies the pulmonary artery as well as the systemic circulation. The pulmonary circulation has a lower vascular resistance (about 3 Wood units) compared to the systemic vascular resistance (about 25 Wood units). This significant difference in resistance will favor blood flow into the pulmonary system leading to excessive pulmonary blood flow and eventual pulmonary edema. The comparatively limited blood flow to the systemic circulation will result in poor systemic cardiac output and, in extreme cases, can manifest as cardiogenic shock.

Atrial septal communication has to be present for survival in these patients.

Pulmonary venous return to the left atrium cannot flow into the left ventricle due to mitral atresia and/or left ventricular hypoplasia. Therefore, blood will cross through an atrial level communication whether a patent foramen ovale (PFO) or an atrial septal defect (ASD), mix with the systemic venous return and pass through the tricuspid valve into the right ventricle.

The phenomenon of pulmonary edema and cardiogenic shock will become more pronounced when the ductus arteriosus starts to close around 2–4 weeks of age. Without an adequate right to left shunt, systemic cardiac output will drop and a right-sided heart failure will develop. The patient will present with severe respiratory distress and poor perfusion evidenced by ashen color, cool extremities, and weak peripheral pulses. Death is imminent unless ductal patency can be maintained, usually with prostaglandin infusion [3, 23 - 25].

RV is the dominant chamber in fetal life transitioning to LV dominance after birth. LV geometry is intended to be the systemic ventricle with its ellipsoid shape and thick walls. On the other hand, RV cavity with its three parts: inlet, apical trabecular and outlet are intended to generate the same cardiac output to the lower vascular resistant pulmonary bed. Therefore RV carries less workload in comparison to LV workload [26, 27].

SV patients with RV morphology were thought to carry higher risk of HF in comparison to those with LV morphologic SV. HLHS is a perfect anatomical example of SV with RV morphology. There have been several studies of the overall outcome post-HLHS staged repair. The presence of right ventricular dysfunction in these patients predicted worse short to midterm outcome post Norwood procedure [28, 29]. There is a debate about whether the morphology of dysfunctional ventricle affects the overall outcome of the single ventricle physiology group [27]. The long term outcome post Fontan completion was found to be similar in patients with functionally single RV compared to patients with functionally single LV and normally related great arteries [30, 31]. On the other hand, the Pediatric Heart Network reported lower EF, diastolic dysfunction and worse exercise performance in patients with systemic RV compared to systemic LV [32, 33]. The true outcome remained to be defined.

In those patients with HLHS, the systemic RV is exposed to chronic volume overload in the early palliative stages that might result in cardiac dilation and myocardial dysfunction. Cardiac dimension and systolic function commonly improve following Fontan procedure [34].

In general, myocardial function in patients post Fontan palliation depends on several factors. The morphology of the systemic ventricle, presence of atriventruiculatr valve regurgitation, type and outcome of early surgical palliative procedures and presence of residual systemic obstructions are some of these factors.

Maintaining normal sinus rhythm and normal conduction in patients with single ventricle are crucial for better outcome after surgical palliation. Unfortunately, this group of patients are more prone to rhythm abnormalities specially atrial arrhythmias leading to myocardial systolic, diastolic or mixed dysfunction [35 - 37]. Every effort has to be taken to re-establish and/or maintain normal sinus rhythm including medications and pacemaker placement (Figs. **6-8**) (Clip 5).

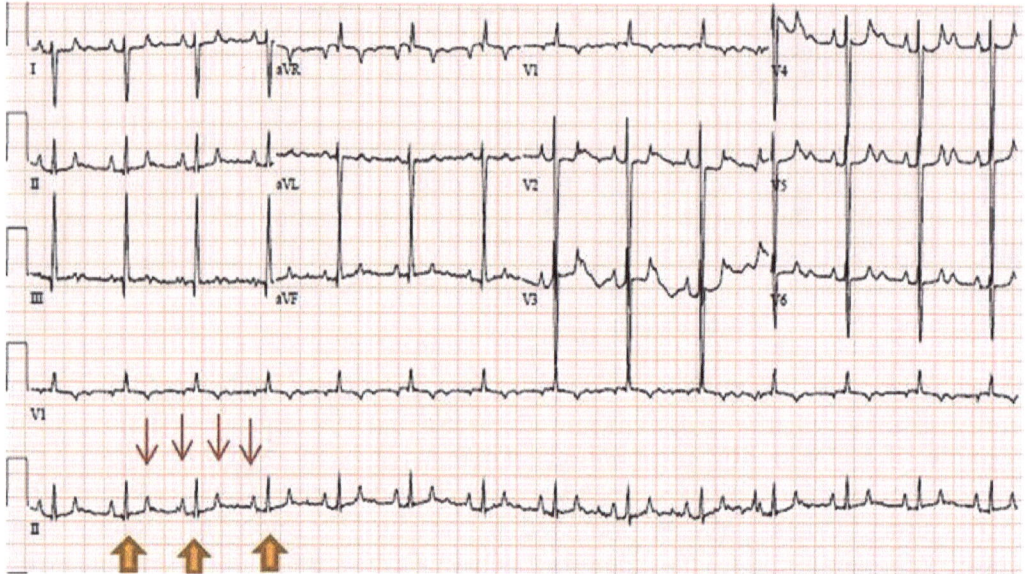

Fig. (6). 12 lead ECG in a one day old female patient with HLHS and a second degree heart block, Mobitz type II. Res arrows points to P waves, orange short arrows point to QRSs.

Manifestations of heart failure following Fontan completion can be subtle. These patients have exercise intolerance at baseline because of the abnormal heart rate response to exercise, in other words chronotropic incompetence [38]. Moreover, exercise related hypoxemia might occur due to residual right to left shunt (in cases of Fenestrated Fontan) or the presence of restrictive lung disease [39].

The presence of ongoing pathological process in certain body organs indicates Fontan failure. Protein loosing enteropathy is the most feared Fontan complication that results from significant congestion of the small intestine leading to poor protein absorption and subsequent protein loss in stools. Liver cirrhosis, plastic bronchitis and renal failure are other significant complications that occur post-surgical palliation of single ventricle patients and carry a high morbidity and mortality risk. Echocardiography and cardiac MRI are used to diagnose failing Fontan, however cardiac catheterization is by far more sensitive tool to evaluate cardiac hemodynamics and diagnose residual defects. Measurement of serum Beta Natriuretic Peptides (BNP) may help identify patients at high risk of heart failure with progressively elevated values in Fontan patients with systemic ventricular failure [32].

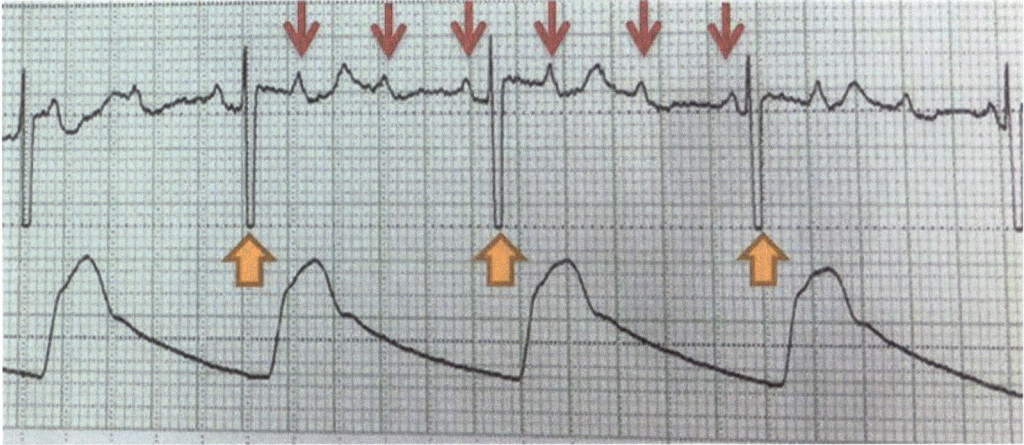

Fig. (7). Rhythm strep with corresponding respiratory movement in the same patient in figure 6 at 2 days of age. Notice the complete dissociation between P waves (red arrows) and QRSs (orange arrows) that indicates third degree heart block.

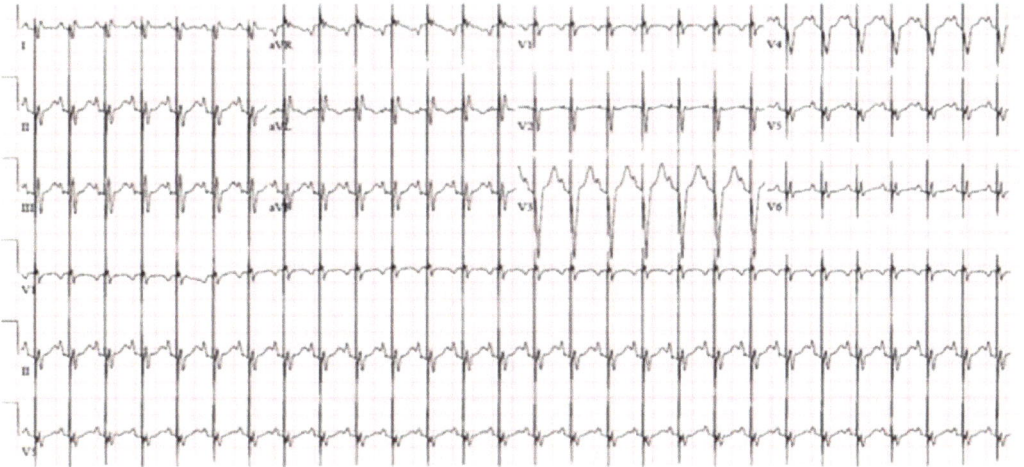

Fig. (8). 12 lead ECG of the same patient in Fig. (**6**) after stage I hybrid procedure and epicardial DDD pacemaker placement at 5 days of age. Please notice the normal sinus rhythm and pacer spikes before every QRS.

Medical treatment in the setting of heart failure in SV patients is a matter of wide debate. The use of angiotensin converting enzyme inhibitors (ACEIs) have been shown to be of no benefit in regard to exercise performance in post Fontan patients [40]. Moreover, in a recent Pediatric Heart Network study, the use of ACEIs before total cavopulmonary shunt showed no difference in somatic growth or ventricular performance compared to patients who were not using ACEIs [2]. B-blockers, particularly Carvedilol, failed to significantly improve heart failure symptoms in SV patients especially those with RV morphology [41].

Definite treatment for patients with failed Fontan remains cardiac transplant. Even that option some times might not be reasonable due to multi-system organ failure in the face of chronically failed Fontan circulation.

Muscular Dystrophy Associated Cardiomyopathy

Muscular dystrophy is a broad classification that describes a group of genetic diseases hallmarked by progressive weakness and associated loss of skeletal muscle mass. While all muscular dystrophies have skeletal muscle involvement, there is a subset that also displays significant cardiac muscle affection. Advances in genetic testing over the past two decades improved our understanding of expected clinical course and outcomes based on particular genetic abnormalities.

Dystrophinopathies, caused by dystrophin deficiency, represent the most common muscular dystrophy with cardiac muscle involvement in childhood. This category includes both Duchenne muscular dystrophy (DMD) and Becker muscular dystrophy (BMD). These dystrophies differ in the type of the dystrophin gene mutation and the resultant expression. Patients with DMD often fail entirely to produce dystrophin and as a result, experience a significantly more severe phenotype. This type is going to be discussed in this chapter as it carries the most significant form of cardiac muscle affection.

Duchenne Muscular Dystrophy

DMD is an X-linked recessive condition that affects approximately 1 in 5,000 male births each year [42]. Previously, patients usually lost their ability to ambulate between 7-13 years of age and only survived to the end of the second or the beginning of the third decade of life. However, the advent of corticosteroid therapy to prolong ambulation combined with dramatic improvements in respiratory support have significantly improved the quality and duration of these patients' lives [43, 44]. With these advances, mortality rates secondary to respiratory failure have declined significantly, and cardiomyopathy and heart failure have emerged as significant causes of morbidity and mortality.

Dystrophin is a protein with significant structural implications, as it directly links the internal cytoskeleton of skeletal and cardiac myocytes to the extracellular matrix. The absence of stabilization typically provided by the dystrophin protein yields significant susceptibility to damage during the mechanical stress of muscle contraction [45]. Absence of the dystrophin protein has also been associated with increases in intracellular calcium, possibly due to perturbation of signaling pathways within the cell. Regardless of the exact etiology, elevated intracellular calcium leads to mitochondrial dysfunction, in turn initiating a profound, uncontrolled inflammatory response [46].

The inflammatory response that ensues from dystrophin deficiency leads to marked fibrosis and fatty replacement of myocardial tissue. Fibrosis typically occurs first in the basal infero-lateral wall of the left ventricle and then expands to include the lateral free wall [47, 48]. With diffuse progression of fibrosis, these patients inevitably develop a generalized dilated cardiomyopathy [44].

Following diagnosis of DMD, cardiac involvement is anticipated, as over 90% of patients will inevitably develop some degree of cardiomyopathy [49, 50]. Therefore, the primary goal of surveillance is early identification in order to ensure early intervention. However, this is particularly challenging in this population, as their limited physical activity often masks symptoms of congestive heart failure that would typically be present.

Echocardiography was the initial noninvasive imaging methodology of choice. It provided visualization of ventricular wall thinning, progression of LV dilation, and significant wall motion abnormalities. However, given the inherent pathophysiology of DMD, a goal of management is to initiate early therapy to reduce or delay the development of fibrotic changes and progression to dilated cardiomyopathy [51]. Therefore, tissue Doppler echocardiography has been utilized in an effort to recognize cardiac dysfunction prior to alterations in ventricular dimensions or development of wall motion abnormalities. Mori *et al*, have identified decreased myocardial velocity gradient during diastole and diminished peak systolic strain as two early indicators of developing cardiomyopathy [52, 53]. However, despite its potential for early detection, echocardiography is often limited by patients' scoliosis and resulting poor acoustic windows.

Strain and strain rate measured by speckle tracking echocardiography (Figs. **2** and **3**) has been used recently for early detection of myocardial dysfunction in DMD patients [54].

As a result of these challenges, cardiac magnetic resonance imaging (CMR) has emerged as a reliable imaging modality to assess ventricular volume, mass, and function. Increased late gadolinium enhancement within the myocardium has also been associated with decreased ejection fraction, and is presumed to represent the initial evidence of fibrosis. Therefore, CMR has the ability to identify one of the earliest markers of cardiac involvement, in turn permitting the earlier institution of protective cardiac therapies [48].

First line therapy for patients with DMD is the early initiation of angiotensin-converting enzyme (ACE) inhibitors. ACE inhibitors reduce peripheral vascular resistance and thus ventricular afterload; as well as reduce ventricular fibrosis and remodeling. A study of DMD patients with an ejection fraction <55%, demonstrated that the initiation of an ACE inhibitor improved cardiac function significantly and delayed further progression of cardiomyopathy [55]. Based on these results and ACE inhibitor's ability to reduce fibrosis formation, a randomized control study was conducted to assess the efficacy of prophylactic ACE inhibitor therapy. At 6 and 10 year follow-up, initiation of ACE inhibitors before the second decade of life and prior to evidence of decreased LV function delayed the onset of LV dysfunction and decreased mortality [56, 57]. As a result, the most recent DMD Working Group Cardiac Care Guidelines recommend initiation of ACE inhibitor therapy by 10 years of age [58].

The second mainstay of therapy for DMD cardiomyopathy is beta blockade. Beta-blockers defer the effects of the sympathetic nervous system, thereby, reducing the cardiac workload and risk of arrhythmia. Multiple studies have demonstrated the benefit of beta blockers in slowing progression to heart failure in patients with DMD [59, 60].

As previously noted, the implementation of glucocorticoid therapy to delay skeletal muscle progression and prolong ambulation has been well documented [61]. In line with this, it has been suggested that prolonged glucocorticoid therapy may be associated with delayed progression of cardiomyopathy as well. One study suggested that continued glucocorticoid treatment led to an overall improvement in morbidity and mortality, primarily related to the deferral of cardiac involvement [62]. Similarly, another study suggested that extended steroid therapy yields delayed cardiac fibrosis as assessed by late gadolinium enhancement on CMR [63]. While each of these studies suggest a promising benefit of glucocorticoid therapy, each is hindered by confounding factors including, homogenous study populations and failure to adequately account for variations in ACE inhibitor, beta-blocker, and aldosterone receptor blockers (ARB) therapy. Due to these confounding variables and the well-documented adverse effects of chronic glucocorticoids, the most recent DMD Working Group Cardiac Care Guidelines does not support the use of prolonged steroid therapy to delay progression of cardiomyopathy [58].

Multiple other therapies have been studied, including proteasome inhibitors [64] and nitric oxide releasing anti-inflammatory agents [65] without significant benefit. Future therapy considerations will be directed at restoring the dystrophin protein within myocytes. Gene therapy currently being pursued is targeting the use of viral vectors to reinstitute functional dystrophin DNA in myocytes [66].

Additionally, stem cell therapies are being explored though have yet to yield any promising modalities to diminish the progression to heart failure.

Left Ventricular Non-Compaction

Left ventricular non-compaction (LVNC) is a heterogeneous myocardial disease first described nine decades ago in 1926, by Grant *et al* [67]. At that time and still today, LVNC has been characterized by three primary criteria: prominent ventricular trabeculations, deep intertrabecular recesses, and the development of two distinct layers of myocardium, compacted and non-compacted [68]. Similar to Grant *et al*'s original case, the majority of early descriptions of LVNC were in association with varying forms of congenital heart disease [69, 70]. However, evidence has emerged that there are patients who reach adulthood without any manifestations of their underlying myocardial anomalies [68].

Insofar that the myocardial manifestations are heterogeneous, the clinical manifestations of the condition are quite varied. However, many patients demonstrate evidence of left ventricular failure, particularly those who present during childhood [71].

During embryonic myocardial development, the ventricles initially exist as a loose meshwork of cardiac muscle fibers. At approximately four weeks gestation, the ventricles begin to develop luminal projections known as trabeculations. These spongy collections of trabeculations serve to increase the surface contact of the ventricular lumen and myocytes as myocardial mass increases prior to the development of the coronary arteries. As the coronary circulation develops from the epicardium to the endocardium, the ventricular myocardium undergoes compaction into organized myocyte bundles from the base to the apex of the heart. Compaction is typically greater in the left ventricle than the right, and is the reason trabeculations are considered a normal aspect of the right ventricular morphology and not that of the left ventricle [72].

Failure to achieve normal compaction may yield significant abnormalities in wall motion and contractile efficacy. The exact etiology of ventricular non-compaction is unclear, though murine and zebrafish models have suggested an association with neuregulin and Notch signaling [73, 74]. Similarly, the precise mechanisms that contribute to progression of heart failure are likely multifactorial. First, myosin ATPase activity is lower in non-compacted myocardium resulting in lower contraction velocity and diminished function [75]. In addition, given the prominence of anomalous trabeculations, there have been hypotheses that microcirculatory anomalies fail to provide adequate perfusion and may yield subendocardial ischemia. This theory is supported by studies, which have demonstrated subendocardial fibrosis on cardiac MRI with late gadolinium enhancement [75]. Potentially further exacerbating this hypoperfusion, non-compacted myocardium is more reliant on aerobic oxidation, and as such is more sensitive to hypoxia [76].

The presentation of LVNC, even in the absence of congenital heart disease, is highly variable. Patients presenting in infancy and early childhood typically do so in congestive heart failure. However, the presentation of patients that reach adolescence and adulthood may range from congestive heart failure to sudden cardiac death to asymptomatic.

A retrospective study performed at Texas Children's Hospital in patients with isolated LVNC found that one-fourth presented with signs and symptoms consistent with congestive heart failure. In addition to congestive heart failure, 17% of patients presented with documented or presumed arrhythmias. This is particularly concerning given that about 12% of those presenting with arrhythmias presented following aborted sudden death. The most common arrhythmias included ventricular tachycardia, atrial tachycardia, and reentrant supraventricular tachycardia [71]. The etiology of the arrhythmogenic myocardium in LVNC is unclear at this time, though may be related to the increased dispersion of repolarization seen in more immature, non-compacted myocardium. In addition to congestive heart failure and arrhythmias, adults often present following a thromboembolic event. 2D and color Doppler, 2 chamber view in a 17 year old presented with syncope and was diagnosed with left ventricular non-compaction. Please notice the deep recesses in the LV apex. In these instances, the lack of laminar flow through intertrabecular recesses combined with stasis caused by a hypokinetic left ventricle are the presumed cause.

Insofar that LVNC is a relatively newly established diagnosis, having only been recognized by the American Heart Association in 2006 [77], there are not yet consensus diagnostic criteria. While echocardiography (Fig. **9**, clip 6) and cardiac MRI are both utilized, echocardiography is typically the initial imaging modality performed. While multiple sets of criteria have been proposed, the most extensively validated and most commonly utilized are those proposed by Jenni, *et al.* [78]. The four criteria include:

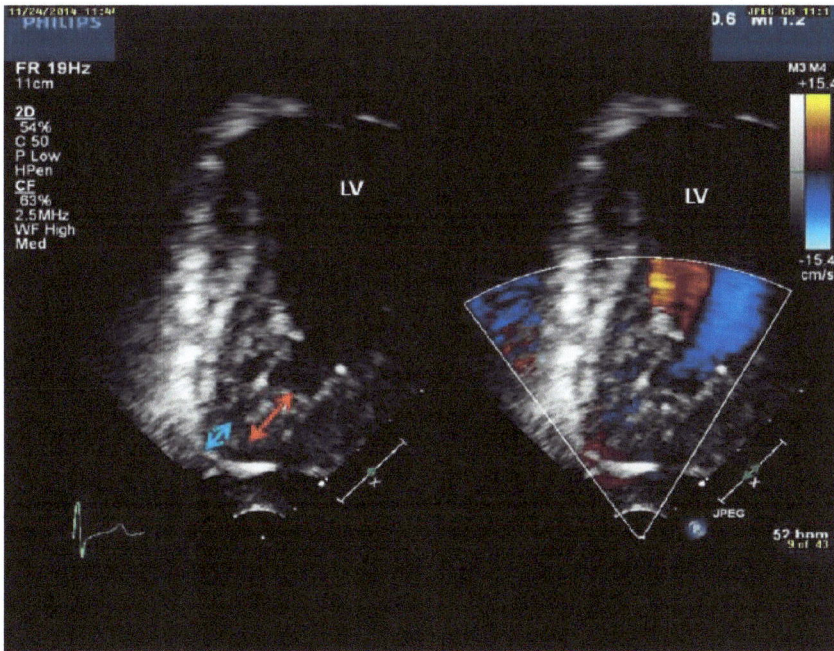

Fig. (9). 2D and color Doppler, 2 chamber view in a 17 year old (same in clip 6) presented with syncope and was diagnosed with left ventricular non-compaction. Please notice the relation between the compacted myocardium (blue double head arrow) and non-compacted myocardium (red double headed arrow).

1. Absence of coexisting cardiac anomalies that would cause the left ventricle to experience excessively high intrauterine pressures so as to predispose to trabeculation formation. These include left outflow tract obstructions or aortic valve obstruction.
2. The presence of two distinct myocardial zones (compacted and non-compacted) with the presence of prominent trabeculations and deep recesses. In addition, the ratio of non-compacted to the compacted myocardium at end-systole must be >2:1.
3. Trabeculations are located at the apical and mid-ventricular segments of the left ventricle and are typically hypokinetic.
4. Color Doppler confirmation of blood flow through the deep intertrabecular recesses.

While the establishment of these criteria has proven helpful in identifying LVNC, echocardiographic visualization of the apex is limited. This may lead to underestimation of the zone of non-compaction and as a result under diagnosis of LVNC. As a result, cardiac MRI has become the imaging modality of choice to confirm a suspected diagnosis. As compared to a ratio of 2:1, a non-compacted to compacted ratio >2.3 has been demonstrated to provide the greatest specificity and sensitivity [79].

Similar to the wide variability in its presentation, LVNC also has multiple phenotypic subtypes. The most commonly described subtypes of isolated LVNC include dilated, hypertrophic, mixed, and those with normal dimensions [71]. Dilated LVNC demonstrates left ventricular dilation with associated systolic dysfunction (Fig. **10**). Hypertrophic LVNC is characterized by left ventricular thickening, with preferential hypertrophy of the septum, and associated diastolic dysfunction. Mixed LVNC demonstrates left ventricular hypertrophy, dilation, and diminished systolic function. This subtype has a higher mortality rate and is more commonly associated with patients with underlying mitochondrial or metabolic diagnoses. Finally, patients with normal ventricular dimensions typically do quite well and have low mortality [71].

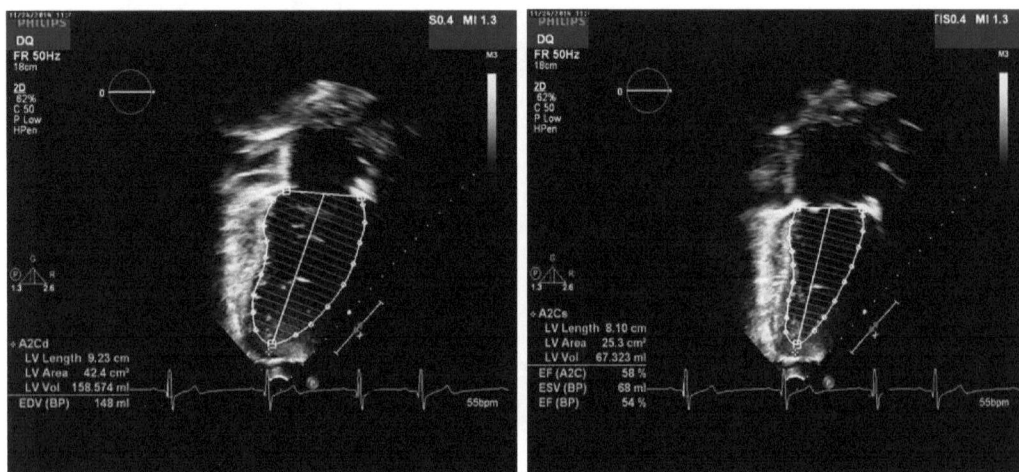

Fig. (10). Same patient in Fig. (**9**) and clip 6. 2D, 2 chamber view with Simpson evaluation of left ventricular systolic function. Please notice border line decreased function with left ventricular ejection fraction (EF) of 54%.

Treatment of patients with LVNC is dependent upon their initial presentation, and for those presenting in heart failure is dependent upon their underlying phenotypic subtype. Guidelines for management are largely extrapolated from those established for other cardiomyopathies contributing to heart failure. Therefore, those with diminished systolic function should be started on beta-blockers and afterload reducing agents such as ACE inhibitors or aldosterone receptor blockers. The latter agents also aid in minimizing ventricular remodeling. It is important to note that there is only one published study regarding the use of beta-blockers in children with LVNC-related systolic dysfunction [80]. Alternatively, patients with a hypertrophic subtype and normal systolic function may benefit from either beta-blockade or calcium channel blockade to minimize hypercontractility and dynamic obstruction within the left ventricle.

In addition to addressing patients' congestive heart failure, therapy should also be focused on minimizing risk of arrhythmias and thromboembolic events. Patients with ventricular tachycardia may benefit from beta blockade alone or might require more aggressive therapy with amiodarone. If these interventions are unsuccessful, implantable cardioverter defibrillators may be considered depending on the patient's age and clinical course. Finally, while thromboembolic events have typically been reported in adult patients, children with dilated atria or left ventricle or significantly decreased ventricular function may benefit from anti-platelet therapy as well.

MANAGEMENT OF HEART FAILURE

Treatment of HF is guided by its etiology. It includes medical, surgical or combination of medical and surgical treatment modalities.

Medical Treatment

Diuretics

Diuretics provide symptomatic relief by reducing intravascular volume and subsequently improved systemic and pulmonary venous congestion. Loop diuretics are considered to be the first line therapy. Nonetheless if loop diuretics are not efficacious, concurrent use of additional diuretic with different mechanism of action, as thiazides diuretics, is often associated with better diuresis. HF activates the Renin-angiotensin-aldosterone system leading to sympathetic activation and accelerated cardiac remodeling. Aldosterone antagonists (AA) like spironolactone and eplerenone are recommended as a corner stone in HF medical management [81].

Angiotensin Converting Enzyme Inhibitors (ACE inhibitors)

ACE inhibitors improve cardiac output through reducing afterload and systolic wall stress. The evidence for its use in pediatric age group was extrapolated from adult literature where ACE inhibitors clearly improved symptoms and reduced mortality in patients with left ventricular systolic dysfunction [82, 83]. In patients with left to right shunt, ACE inhibitors improved growth in some children but caused renal insufficiency when used in premature infants [84]. In another study in patients with SV, Enalapril, as an example of ACE inhibitor, did not improve somatic growth, ventricular function, or severity of HF when administered in the first year of life [85]. ACE inhibitors reduced the amount of pleural drainage and its duration when given in the perioperative period in Glenn patients [86]. On the other hand, Enalapril effect on the cardiac output in Glenn patients was not significant despite its role in decreasing the systemic vascular resistant. Instead, it was noticed to cause reduction in the arterial oxygen saturation *via* redistribution of the flow in the lower body [87].

Angiotensin Receptor Blockers (ARBs)

There are limited data available on its use in children, so it is not going to be discussed in this chapter.

Digoxin

Digoxin is a Na/K ATPase inhibitor and has multiple effects on the cardiovascular system including improvement of myocardial contractility, a decrease in sympathetic signals and an increase in vagal tone together with a decrease in serum norepinephrine. As old of a medication as it is, many cardiologists still prefer to use it in treatment of arrhythmias and HF symptoms. Due to its narrow therapeutic index, its role in HF treatment became less prominent and a matter of debate. Studies had showed lack of survival rate improvement in adult patients with HF [88]. Some other studies found a beneficial effect in patients with large left to right shunt [89]. On the other hand, many studies do not support its use in patients with large shunts owing to its effect on augmenting pulmonary flow [90].

Beta-blockers

Beta-blockers (*e.g.* Metoprolol and Carvedilol) were found to have a beneficial effect in adult patients with heart failure [91, 92]. There are several proposed explanations of such effect [93]:

1. Reduction of excessive adrenergic stimulation of the myocardium.
2. Induction of slower heart rate and lower blood pressure
3. Inhibition of renin-angiotensin system
4. Antiarrhythmic properties
5. Antioxidant effect.

Few studies suggested beneficial effect of B blockers in treatment of children with chronic HF [94], DMD [60] and following chemotherapy [95]. The Pediatric Carvedilol trial showed no significant effect of Carvedilol compared to placebo on the clinical HF outcome. However, it suggested a beneficial effect in HF symptoms in SV patients who have LV morphologic SV compared to RV morphology [41].

Anticoagulation

Patients with HF are at increased risk of thromboembolism compared to patients with normal ventricular function. The risk increases with increased degree of myocardial dysfunction. Administration of anticoagulation medications is strongly suggested. The regimen varies between use of Aspirin in moderately depressed cardiac function to Warfarin or Enoxaparin in severe forms of HF and significantly depressed myocardial function.

The epidemiology of thromboembolism in paediatric patients differs widely from adults [96, 97].

The development of haemostatic system in children can affect their response to anticoagulants [98].

In addition, the pharmacokinetics of antithrombotic drugs are age-dependent [99].

Therefore, the successful use of anticoagulation in paediatric patients requires a collaborative team [100].

Family and patient contribution is also very essential due to limited vascular access, lack of comprehension and co-operation of the child and other tolerability issues that reduces the ability to effectively deliver anticoagulation drugs [101].

The commonly used anticoagulants in pediatric populations are: vitamin K antagonist, unfractionated heparin and Low molecular weight heparins (LMWH).

LMWHs have rapidly been the drug of choice for prophylaxis and treatment of thromboembolism in pediatric patients. Their efficacy, however, has not been yet proven. There is still no enough data about the use of novel anticoagulants in pediatric populations [101].

CONCLUSION

Heart failure in pediatric populations has many causes. Congenital heart disease is one of causes in heart failure in this group. Congenital cardiomyopathy, single ventricle and Fallot tetralogy are some of causes of heart failure in infants and children. Echocardiography and catheterization can help diagnosis and directing the management. Medical treatment as diuretics, ACE inhibitors iand digoxin should be started before proceeding to interventional or surgical treatment.

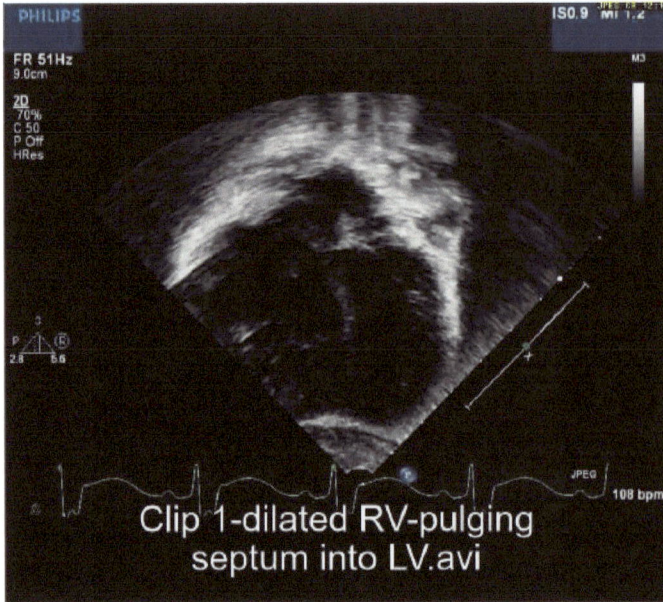

Clip (1). Dilated RV-pulging septum into LV.
Link: https://vimeo.com/380652522
Password: eurekac6af18

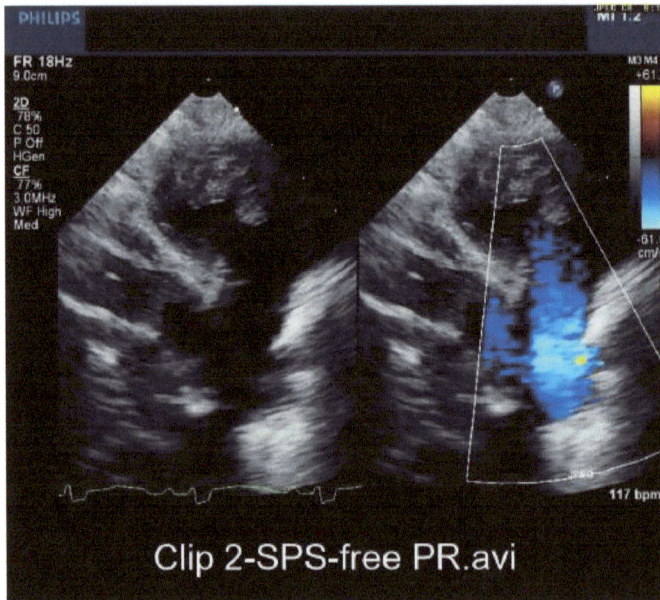

Clip (2). SPS-free PR.
Link: https://vimeo.com/380676489
Password: eurekac6af18

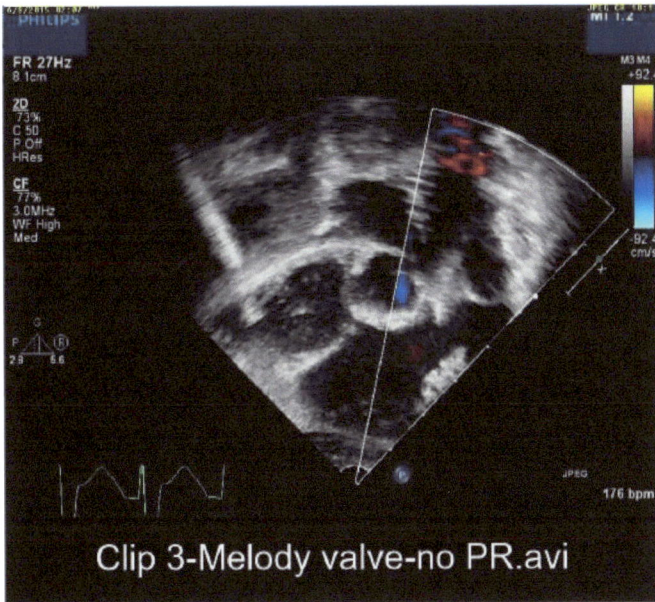

Clip (3). Melody valve-no PR.
Link: https://vimeo.com/380677851
Password: eurekac6af18

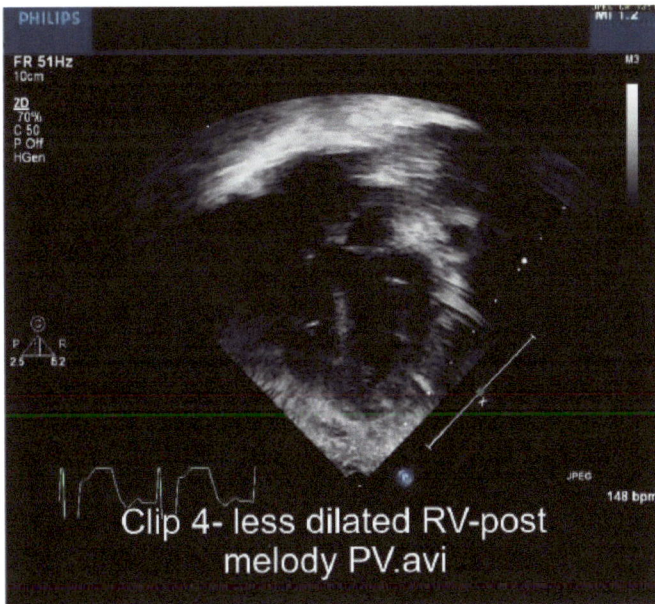

Clip (4). Less dilated RV-post melody PV.
Link: https://vimeo.com/380678746
Password: eurekac6af18

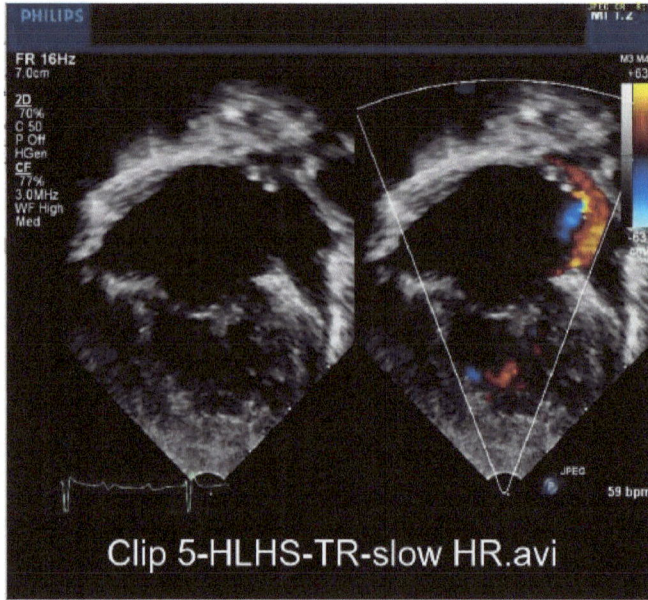

Clip (5). HLHS-TR-slow HR.
Link: https://vimeo.com/380679244
Password: eurekac6af18

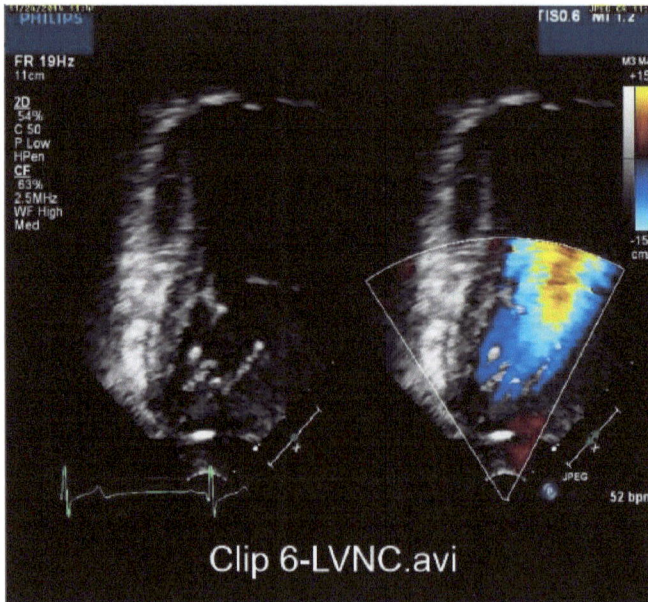

Clip (6). LVNC.
Link: https://vimeo.com/380679548
Password: eurekac6af18

CONSENT FOR PUBLICATION

Not applicable.

CONFLICT OF INTEREST

The authors confirm that this chapter contents have no conflict of interest.

ACKNOWLEDGEMENTS

Declared none.

REFERENCES

[1]   Rossano JW, Shaddy RE. Heart failure in children: etiology and treatment. J Pediatr 2014; 165(2): 228-33.http://www.ncbi.nlm.nih.gov/pubmed/24928699 [Internet].
        [http://dx.doi.org/10.1016/j.jpeds.2014.04.055] [PMID: 24928699]

[2]   Hsu DT, Pearson GD. Heart failure in children: part II: diagnosis, treatment, and future directions. Circ Heart Fail 2009; 2(5): 490-8.
        [http://dx.doi.org/10.1161/CIRCHEARTFAILURE.109.856229] [PMID: 19808380]

[3]   Hsu DT, Pearson GD. Heart failure in children: part I: history, etiology, and pathophysiology. Circ Heart Fail 2009; 2(1): 63-70.
        [http://dx.doi.org/10.1161/CIRCHEARTFAILURE.108.820217] [PMID: 19808316]

[4]   Watson DG, Smith JC, Warren ET. Congestive heart failure with tetralogy of Fallot relieved by an aortopulmonary shunt. Pediatr Cardiol 1997; 18(5): 381-4.
        [http://dx.doi.org/10.1007/s002469900206] [PMID: 9270111]

[5]   Ogunkunle OO, Omokhodion SI, Oladokun RE, Odutola AA. Heart failure complicating tetralogy of Fallot. West Afr J Med 2004; 23(1): 75-8.
        [http://dx.doi.org/10.4314/wajm.v23i1.28089] [PMID: 15171534]

[6]   Wessel HU, Paul MH. Exercise studies in tetralogy of Fallot: a review. Pediatr Cardiol 1999; 20(1): 39-47.
        [http://dx.doi.org/10.1007/s002469900393] [PMID: 9861075]

[7]   Mahle WT, Parks WJ, Fyfe DA, Sallee D. Tricuspid regurgitation in patients with repaired Tetralogy of Fallot and its relation to right ventricular dilatation. Am J Cardiol 2003; 92(5): 643-5.
        [http://dx.doi.org/10.1016/S0002-9149(03)00746-X] [PMID: 12943899]

[8]   Babu-Narayan SV, Kilner PJ, Li W, et al. Ventricular fibrosis suggested by cardiovascular magnetic resonance in adults with repaired tetralogy of fallot and its relationship to adverse markers of clinical outcome. Circulation 2006; 113(3): 405-13.
        [http://dx.doi.org/10.1161/CIRCULATIONAHA.105.548727] [PMID: 16432072]

[9]   Norgård G, Gatzoulis MA, Josen M, Cullen S, Redington AN. Does restrictive right ventricular physiology in the early postoperative period predict subsequent right ventricular restriction after repair of tetralogy of Fallot? Heart 1998; 79(5): 481-4.
        [http://dx.doi.org/10.1136/hrt.79.5.481] [PMID: 9659195]

[10]   Friedberg MK, Fernandes FP, Roche SL, et al. Impaired right and left ventricular diastolic myocardial mechanics and filling in asymptomatic children and adolescents after repair of tetralogy of Fallot. Eur Heart J Cardiovasc Imaging 2012; 13(11): 905-13.
        [http://dx.doi.org/10.1093/ehjci/jes067] [PMID: 22467442]

[11]   Hugh D. Allen MD , David J. Driscoll MD , Robert E. Shaddy TFF. Moss & Adams' Heart Disease in Infants, Children, and Adolescents: Including the Fetus and Young Adult. 8th ed. Philadelphia: LWW;

Eighth; 2013. 981-984 p

[12] Gatzoulis MA, Till JA, Somerville J, Redington AN. Mechanoelectrical interaction in tetralogy of Fallot. QRS prolongation relates to right ventricular size and predicts malignant ventricular arrhythmias and sudden death. Circulation 1995; 92(2): 231-7.
[http://dx.doi.org/10.1161/01.CIR.92.2.231] [PMID: 7600655]

[13] Helbing WA, Niezen RA, Le Cessie S, van der Geest RJ, Ottenkamp J, de Roos A. Right ventricular diastolic function in children with pulmonary regurgitation after repair of tetralogy of Fallot: volumetric evaluation by magnetic resonance velocity mapping. J Am Coll Cardiol 1996; 28(7): 1827-35.
[http://dx.doi.org/10.1016/S0735-1097(96)00387-7] [PMID: 8962573]

[14] Tzemos N, Harris L, Carasso S, et al. Adverse left ventricular mechanics in adults with repaired tetralogy of Fallot. Am J Cardiol 2009; 103(3): 420-5.
[http://dx.doi.org/10.1016/j.amjcard.2008.09.101] [PMID: 19166701]

[15] Geva T, Sandweiss BM, Gauvreau K, Lock JE, Powell AJ. Factors associated with impaired clinical status in long-term survivors of tetralogy of Fallot repair evaluated by magnetic resonance imaging. J Am Coll Cardiol 2004; 43(6): 1068-74.
[http://dx.doi.org/10.1016/j.jacc.2003.10.045] [PMID: 15028368]

[16] Ghai A, Silversides C, Harris L, Webb GD, Siu SC, Therrien J. Left ventricular dysfunction is a risk factor for sudden cardiac death in adults late after repair of tetralogy of Fallot. J Am Coll Cardiol 2002; 40(9): 1675-80.
[http://dx.doi.org/10.1016/S0735-1097(02)02344-6] [PMID: 12427422]

[17] Kane C, Kogon B, Pernetz M, et al. Left ventricular function improves after pulmonary valve replacement in patients with previous right ventricular outflow tract reconstruction and biventricular dysfunction. Tex Heart Inst J 2011; 38(3): 234-7.
[PMID: 21720459]

[18] Raman SV, Cook SC, McCarthy B, Ferketich AK. Usefulness of multidetector row computed tomography to quantify right ventricular size and function in adults with either tetralogy of Fallot or transposition of the great arteries. Am J Cardiol 2005; 95(5): 683-6.
[http://dx.doi.org/10.1016/j.amjcard.2004.11.014] [PMID: 15721122]

[19] Babu-Narayan SV, Uebing A, Davlouros PA, et al. Randomised trial of ramipril in repaired tetralogy of Fallot and pulmonary regurgitation: the APPROPRIATE study (Ace inhibitors for Potential PRevention Of the deleterious effects of Pulmonary Regurgitation In Adults with repaired TEtralogy of Fallot). Int J Cardiol 2012; 154(3): 299-305.
[http://dx.doi.org/10.1016/j.ijcard.2010.09.057] [PMID: 20970202]

[20] Norozi K, Bahlmann J, Raab B, Alpers V, Arnhold JO, Kuehne T, et al. A prospective, randomized, double-blind, placebo controlled trial of beta-blockade in patients who have undergone surgical correction of tetralogy of Fallot. Cardiol Young [Internet] 17(4):372–9. Available from: http://www.embase.com/search/results?subaction=viewrecord&from=export&id=L47215367
[http://dx.doi.org/10.1017/S1047951107000844]

[21] Kaulitz R, Hofbeck M. Current treatment and prognosis in children with functionally univentricular hearts. Arch Dis Child 2005; 90(7): 757-62.
[http://dx.doi.org/10.1136/adc.2003.034090] [PMID: 15970622]

[22] Khairy P, Poirier N, Mercier LA. Univentricular heart. Circulation 2007; 115(6): 800-12.
[http://dx.doi.org/10.1161/CIRCULATIONAHA.105.592378] [PMID: 17296869]

[23] Abdulla R. Heart Diseases in Children [Internet]. Boston, MA: Springer US; 2011. 273-282 p. Available from: http://link.springer.com/10.1007/978-1-4419-7994-0

[24] Feinstein JA, Benson DW, Dubin AM, et al. Hypoplastic left heart syndrome: current considerations and expectations. J Am Coll Cardiol 2012; 59(1) (Suppl.): S1-S42.
[http://dx.doi.org/10.1016/j.jacc.2011.09.022] [PMID: 22192720]

[25]   Shaddy RE. Heart Failure in Congenital Heart Disease: [Internet]. first edit. Shaddy RE, editor. London: Springer   London;   2011.   30-37   p.   Available   from: http://link.springer.com/10.1007/978-1-84996-480-7

[26]   Dell'Italia LJ. Anatomy and physiology of the right ventricle. Cardiol Clin 2012; 30(2): 167-87.http://www.ncbi.nlm.nih.gov/pubmed/22548810 [Internet].
[http://dx.doi.org/10.1016/j.ccl.2012.03.009] [PMID: 22548810]

[27]   Roche SL, Redington AN. The failing right ventricle in congenital heart disease. Can J Cardiol 2013; 29(7): 768-78.http://www.ncbi.nlm.nih.gov/pubmed/23790549 [Internet].
[http://dx.doi.org/10.1016/j.cjca.2013.04.018] [PMID: 23790549]

[28]   Altmann K, Printz BF, Solowiejczky DE, Gersony WM, Quaegebeur J, Apfel HD. Two-dimensional echocardiographic assessment of right ventricular function as a predictor of outcome in hypoplastic left heart syndrome. Am J Cardiol 2000; 86(9): 964-8.
[http://dx.doi.org/10.1016/S0002-9149(00)01131-0] [PMID: 11053708]

[29]   Walsh MA, McCrindle BW, Dipchand A, *et al.* Left ventricular morphology influences mortality after the Norwood operation. Heart 2009; 95(15): 1238-44.
[http://dx.doi.org/10.1136/hrt.2008.156612] [PMID: 19457871]

[30]   Gaynor JW, Bridges ND, Cohen MI, *et al.* Predictors of outcome after the Fontan operation: is hypoplastic left heart syndrome still a risk factor? J Thorac Cardiovasc Surg 2002; 123(2): 237-45.http://linkinghub.elsevier.com/retrieve/pii/S0022522302501872 [Internet].
[http://dx.doi.org/10.1067/mtc.2002.119337] [PMID: 11828282]

[31]   Gentles TL, Mayer JE Jr, Gauvreau K, *et al.* Fontan operation in five hundred consecutive patients: factors influencing early and late outcome. J Thorac Cardiovasc Surg 1997; 114(3): 376-91.
[http://dx.doi.org/10.1016/S0022-5223(97)70183-1] [PMID: 9305190]

[32]   Anderson PAW, Sleeper LA, Mahony L, *et al.* Contemporary outcomes after the Fontan procedure: a Pediatric Heart Network multicenter study. J Am Coll Cardiol 2008; 52(2): 85-98.
[http://dx.doi.org/10.1016/j.jacc.2008.01.074] [PMID: 18598886]

[33]   Paridon SM, Mitchell PD, Colan SD, *et al.* A cross-sectional study of exercise performance during the first 2 decades of life after the Fontan operation. J Am Coll Cardiol 2008; 52(2): 99-107.
[http://dx.doi.org/10.1016/j.jacc.2008.02.081] [PMID: 18598887]

[34]   Sluysmans T, Sanders SP, van der Velde M, *et al.* Natural history and patterns of recovery of contractile function in single left ventricle after Fontan operation. Circulation 1992; 86(6): 1753-61.
[http://dx.doi.org/10.1161/01.CIR.86.6.1753] [PMID: 1451247]

[35]   Ghai A, Harris L, Harrison DA, Webb GD, Siu SC. Outcomes of late atrial tachyarrhythmias in adults after the Fontan operation. J Am Coll Cardiol 2001; 37(2): 585-92.
[http://dx.doi.org/10.1016/S0735-1097(00)01141-4] [PMID: 11216983]

[36]   Cheung YF, Penny DJ, Redington AN. Serial assessment of left ventricular diastolic function after Fontan procedure. Heart 2000; 83(4): 420-4.
[http://dx.doi.org/10.1136/heart.83.4.420] [PMID: 10722541]

[37]   Mahle WT, Coon PD, Wernovsky G, Rychik J. Quantitative echocardiographic assessment of the performance of the functionally single right ventricle after the Fontan operation. Cardiol Young 2001; 11(4): 399-406.
[http://dx.doi.org/10.1017/S1047951101000518] [PMID: 11558949]

[38]   Diller G-P, Dimopoulos K, Okonko D, *et al.* Heart rate response during exercise predicts survival in adults   with   congenital   heart   disease.   J   Am   Coll   Cardiol   2006;   48(6): 1250-6.http://www.ncbi.nlm.nih.gov/pubmed/16979014 [Internet].
[http://dx.doi.org/10.1016/j.jacc.2006.05.051] [PMID: 16979014]

[39]   Rosenthal D, Chrisant MRK, Edens E, *et al.* International Society for Heart and Lung Transplantation: Practice guidelines for management of heart failure in children. J Heart Lung Transplant 2004; 23(12):

1313-33.
[http://dx.doi.org/10.1016/j.healun.2004.03.018] [PMID: 15607659]

[40] Kouatli AA, Garcia JA, Zellers TM, Weinstein EM, Mahony L. Enalapril does not enhance exercise capacity in patients after Fontan procedure. Circulation 1997; 96(5): 1507-12.
[http://dx.doi.org/10.1161/01.CIR.96.5.1507] [PMID: 9315539]

[41] Shaddy RE, Boucek MM, Hsu DT, *et al.* Carvedilol for children and adolescents with heart failure: a randomized controlled trial. JAMA 2007; 298(10): 1171-9.
[http://dx.doi.org/10.1001/jama.298.10.1171] [PMID: 17848651]

[42] Alberta HR. Prevalence of Duchenne/Becker muscular dystrophy among males aged 5-24 years - four states, 2007. MMWR Morb Mortal Wkly Rep 2009; 58(40): 1119-22.
[PMID: 19834452]

[43] Wong BLY, Christopher C. Corticosteroids in Duchenne muscular dystrophy: a reappraisal. J Child Neurol 2002; 17(3): 183-90.
[http://dx.doi.org/10.1177/088307380201700306] [PMID: 12026233]

[44] Eagle M, Baudouin SV, Chandler C, Giddings DR, Bullock R, Bushby K. Survival in Duchenne muscular dystrophy: improvements in life expectancy since 1967 and the impact of home nocturnal ventilation. Neuromuscul Disord 2002; 12(10): 926-9.
[http://dx.doi.org/10.1016/S0960-8966(02)00140-2] [PMID: 12467747]

[45] Blake DJ, Weir A, Newey SE, Davies KE. Function and genetics of dystrophin and dystrophin-related proteins in muscle. Physiol Rev 2002; 82(2): 291-329.
[http://dx.doi.org/10.1152/physrev.00028.2001] [PMID: 11917091]

[46] Altamirano F, López JR, Henríquez C, Molinski T, Allen PD, Jaimovich E. Increased resting intracellular calcium modulates NF-κB-dependent inducible nitric-oxide synthase gene expression in dystrophic mdx skeletal myotubes. J Biol Chem 2012; 287(25): 20876-87.
[http://dx.doi.org/10.1074/jbc.M112.344929] [PMID: 22549782]

[47] Sasaki K, Sakata K, Kachi E, Hirata S, Ishihara T, Ishikawa K. Sequential changes in cardiac structure and function in patients with Duchenne type muscular dystrophy: a two-dimensional echocardiographic study. Am Heart J 1998; 135(6 Pt 1): 937-44.
[http://dx.doi.org/10.1016/S0002-8703(98)70057-2] [PMID: 9630096]

[48] Puchalski MD, Williams RV, Askovich B, *et al.* Late gadolinium enhancement: precursor to cardiomyopathy in Duchenne muscular dystrophy? Int J Cardiovasc Imaging 2009; 25(1): 57-63.
[http://dx.doi.org/10.1007/s10554-008-9352-y] [PMID: 18686011]

[49] Finsterer J, Stöllberger C. The heart in human dystrophinopathies. Cardiology 2003; 99(1): 1-19.
[http://dx.doi.org/10.1159/000068446] [PMID: 12589117]

[50] Nigro G, Comi LI, Politano L, Bain RJI. The incidence and evolution of cardiomyopathy in Duchenne muscular dystrophy. Int J Cardiol 1990; 26(3): 271-7.
[http://dx.doi.org/10.1016/0167-5273(90)90082-G] [PMID: 2312196]

[51] Surgery C. Cardiovascular health supervision for individuals affected by Duchenne or Becker muscular dystrophy. Pediatrics 2005; 116(6): 1569-73.
[http://dx.doi.org/10.1542/peds.2005-2448] [PMID: 16322188]

[52] Mori K, Edagawa T, Inoue M, *et al.* Peak negative myocardial velocity gradient and wall-thickening velocity during early diastole are noninvasive parameters of left ventricular diastolic function in patients with Duchenne's progressive muscular dystrophy. J Am Soc Echocardiogr 2004; 17(4): 322-9.
[http://dx.doi.org/10.1016/j.echo.2003.12.016] [PMID: 15044864]

[53] Mori K, Hayabuchi Y, Inoue M, Suzuki M, Sakata M, Nakagawa R, *et al.* Myocardial strain imaging for early detection of cardiac involvement in patients with Duchenne's progressive muscular dystrophy. Echocardiography [Internet]. 2007 Jul [cited 2015 Jan 12];24(6):598–608. Available from: http://www.ncbi.nlm.nih.gov/pubmed/17584199

[http://dx.doi.org/10.1111/j.1540-8175.2007.00437.x]

[54]   Ryan TD, Taylor MD, Mazur W, Cripe LH, Pratt J, King EC, *et al.* Abnormal circumferential strain is present in young Duchenne muscular dystrophy patients. Pediatr Cardiol [Internet]. 2013 Jun [cited 2015 Jan 12];34(5):1159–65. Available from: http://www.ncbi.nlm.nih.gov/pubmed/23358912
       [http://dx.doi.org/10.1007/s00246-012-0622-z]

[55]   Viollet L, Thrush PT, Flanigan KM, Mendell JR, Allen HD. Effects of angiotensin-converting enzyme inhibitors and/or beta blockers on the cardiomyopathy in Duchenne muscular dystrophy. Am J Cardiol 2012; 110(1): 98-102.
       [http://dx.doi.org/10.1016/j.amjcard.2012.02.064] [PMID: 22463839]

[56]   Duboc D, Meune C, Lerebours G, Devaux J-Y, Vaksmann G, Bécane H-M. 2005. Mar 15 [cited 2015 Jan 20];45(6):855–7. Available from: http://www.ncbi.nlm.nih.gov/pubmed/15766818

[57]   Duboc D, Meune C, Pierre B, *et al.* Perindopril preventive treatment on mortality in Duchenne muscular dystrophy: 10 years' follow-up. Am Heart J 2007; 154(3): 596-602.
       [http://dx.doi.org/10.1016/j.ahj.2007.05.014] [PMID: 17719312]

[58]   McNally EM, Kaltman JR, Benson DW, *et al.* Contemporary cardiac issues in Duchenne muscular dystrophy. Working Group of the National Heart, Lung, and Blood Institute in collaboration with Parent   Project   Muscular   Dystrophy.   Circulation   2015;   131(18): 1590-8.http://circ.ahajournals.org/cgi/doi/10.1161/CIRCULATIONAHA.114.015151 [Internet].
       [http://dx.doi.org/10.1161/CIRCULATIONAHA.114.015151] [PMID: 25940966]

[59]   Ogata H, Ishikawa Y, Ishikawa Y, Minami R. Beneficial effects of beta-blockers and angiotensin-converting enzyme inhibitors in Duchenne muscular dystrophy. J Cardiol 2009; 53(1): 72-8.
       [http://dx.doi.org/10.1016/j.jjcc.2008.08.013] [PMID: 19167641]

[60]   Kajimoto H, Ishigaki K, Okumura K, *et al.* Beta-blocker therapy for cardiac dysfunction in patients with muscular dystrophy. Circ J 2006; 70(8): 991-4.
       [http://dx.doi.org/10.1253/circj.70.991] [PMID: 16864930]

[61]   Manzur AY, Kuntzer T, Pike M, Swan A. Glucocorticoid corticosteroids for Duchenne muscular dystrophy. Cochrane Database Syst Rev 2008; (1): CD003725
       [PMID: 18254031]

[62]   Schram G, Fournier A, Leduc H, *et al.* All-cause mortality and cardiovascular outcomes with prophylactic steroid therapy in Duchenne muscular dystrophy. J Am Coll Cardiol 2013; 61(9): 948-54.
       [http://dx.doi.org/10.1016/j.jacc.2012.12.008] [PMID: 23352781]

[63]   Tandon a. Villa CR, Hor KN, Jefferies JL, Gao Z, Towbin J a., *et al.* Myocardial Fibrosis Burden Predicts Left Ventricular Ejection Fraction and Is Associated With Age and Steroid Treatment Duration in Duchenne Muscular Dystrophy. J Am Heart Assoc [Internet]. 2015; 4(4): e001338–e001338. Available from: http://jaha. ahajournals. org/ cgi/ doi/10.1161/JAHA.114.0013 38

[64]   Bonuccelli G, Sotgia F, Schubert W, *et al.* Proteasome inhibitor (MG-132) treatment of mdx mice rescues the expression and membrane localization of dystrophin and dystrophin-associated proteins. Am J Pathol 2003; 163(4): 1663-75.
       [http://dx.doi.org/10.1016/S0002-9440(10)63523-7] [PMID: 14507673]

[65]   Brunelli S, Sciorati C, D'Antona G, *et al.* Nitric oxide release combined with nonsteroidal antiinflammatory activity prevents muscular dystrophy pathology and enhances stem cell therapy. Proc Natl Acad Sci USA 2007; 104(1): 264-9.
       [http://dx.doi.org/10.1073/pnas.0608277104] [PMID: 17182743]

[66]   Bostick B, Yue Y, Long C, *et al.* Cardiac expression of a mini-dystrophin that normalizes skeletal muscle force only partially restores heart function in aged Mdx mice. Mol Ther 2009; 17(2): 253-61.
       [http://dx.doi.org/10.1038/mt.2008.264] [PMID: 19066599]

[67]   Medicine C, Floria M, Tinica G, Grecu M, Popa GT. Left ventricular non-compaction – challenges and controversies 2014; 9(3): 282-8.

[68] Chin TK, Perloff JK, Williams RG, Jue K, Mohrmann R. Isolated noncompaction of left ventricular myocardium. A study of eight cases. Circulation 1990; 82(2): 507-13.
[http://dx.doi.org/10.1161/01.CIR.82.2.507] [PMID: 2372897]

[69] Stähli BE, Gebhard C, Biaggi P, *et al.* Left ventricular non-compaction: prevalence in congenital heart disease. Int J Cardiol 2013; 167(6): 2477-81.
[http://dx.doi.org/10.1016/j.ijcard.2012.05.095] [PMID: 22704867]

[70] Towbin JA. Left ventricular noncompaction: a new form of heart failure. Heart Fail Clin 2010; 6(4): 453-469, viii.
[http://dx.doi.org/10.1016/j.hfc.2010.06.005] [PMID: 20869646]

[71] Brescia ST, Rossano JW, Pignatelli R, *et al.* Mortality and sudden death in pediatric left ventricular noncompaction in a tertiary referral center. Circulation 2013; 127(22): 2202-8.
[http://dx.doi.org/10.1161/CIRCULATIONAHA.113.002511] [PMID: 23633270]

[72] Sedmera D, McQuinn T. Embryogenesis of the heart muscle. Heart Fail Clin 2008; 4(3): 235-45.
[http://dx.doi.org/10.1016/j.hfc.2008.02.007] [PMID: 18598977]

[73] Meyer D, Birchmeier C. Multiple essential functions of neuregulin in development. Nature 1995; 378(6555): 386-90.
[http://dx.doi.org/10.1038/378386a0] [PMID: 7477375]

[74] Luxán G, Casanova JC, Martínez-Poveda B, *et al.* Mutations in the NOTCH pathway regulator MIB1 cause left ventricular noncompaction cardiomyopathy. Nat Med 2013; 19(2): 193-201.http://www. ncbi. nlm. nih. gov/pubmed/23314057 [Internet].
[http://dx.doi.org/10.1038/nm.3046] [PMID: 23314 057]

[75] Hamamichi Y, Ichida F, Hashimoto I, *et al.* Isolated noncompaction of the ventricular myocardium: ultrafast computed tomography and magnetic resonance imaging. Int J Cardiovasc Imaging 2001; 17(4): 305-14.
[http://dx.doi.org/10.1023/A:1011658926555] [PMID: 11599870]

[76] Oštádal B. Comparative Aspects of the Cardiac Blood Supply. Adv Organ Biol 1999; 7(C): 91-110.
[http://dx.doi.org/10.1016/S1569-2590(08)60164-0]

[77] Maron BJ, Towbin JA, Thiene G, *et al.* American Heart Association; Council on Clinical Cardiology, Heart Failure and Transplantation Committee; Quality of Care and Outcomes Research and Functional Genomics and Translational Biology Interdisciplinary Working Groups; Council on Epidemiology and Prevention. Contemporary definitions and classification of the cardiomyopathies: an American Heart Association Scientific Statement from the Council on Clinical Cardiology, Heart Failure and Transplantation Committee; Quality of Care and Outcomes Research and Functional Genomics and Translational Biology Interdisciplinary Working Groups; and Council on Epidemiology and Prevention. Circulation 2006; 113(14): 1807-16.http://circ.ahajournals.org/content/113/14/1807 [Internet].
[http://dx.doi.org/10.1161/CIRCULATIONAHA.106.174287] [PMID: 16567565]

[78] Jenni R, Oechslin E, Schneider J, Attenhofer Jost C, Kaufmann PA. Echocardiographic and pathoanatomical characteristics of isolated left ventricular non-compaction: a step towards classification as a distinct cardiomyopathy. Heart 2001; 86(6): 666-71.
[http://dx.doi.org/10.1136/heart.86.6.666] [PMID: 11711464]

[79] Petersen SE, Selvanayagam JB, Wiesmann F, *et al.* Left ventricular non-compaction: insights from cardiovascular magnetic resonance imaging. J Am Coll Cardiol 2005; 46(1): 101-5.
[http://dx.doi.org/10.1016/j.jacc.2005.03.045] [PMID: 15992642]

[80] Toyono M, Kondo C, Nakajima Y, Nakazawa M, Momma K, Kusakabe K. Effects of carvedilol on left ventricular function, mass, and scintigraphic findings in isolated left ventricular non-compaction. Heart 2001; 86(1)E4
[http://dx.doi.org/10.1136/heart.86.1.e4] [PMID: 11410581]

[81] Tsutamoto T, Wada A, Maeda K, *et al.* Effect of spironolactone on plasma brain natriuretic peptide and left ventricular remodeling in patients with congestive heart failure. J Am Coll Cardiol 2001; 37(5): 1228-33.
[http://dx.doi.org/10.1016/S0735-1097(01)01116-0] [PMID: 11300427]

[82] Garg R, Yusuf S. Overview of randomized trials of angiotensin-converting enzyme inhibitors on mortality and morbidity in patients with heart failure. JAMA 1995; 273(18): 1450-6.
[http://dx.doi.org/10.1001/jama.1995.03520420066040] [PMID: 7654275]

[83] Yusuf S, Pitt B, Davis CE, Hood WB, Cohn JN. Effect of enalapril on survival in patients with reduced left ventricular ejection fractions and congestive heart failure. N Engl J Med 1991; 325(5): 293-302.http://www.ncbi.nlm.nih.gov/pubmed/2057034 [Internet].
[http://dx.doi.org/10.1056/NEJM199108013250501] [PMID: 2057034]

[84] Book WM. Heart failure in the adult patient with congenital heart disease. J Card Fail 2005; 11(4): 306-12.
[http://dx.doi.org/10.1016/j.cardfail.2004.08.162] [PMID: 15880341]

[85] Hsu DT, Zak V, Mahony L, *et al.* Enalapril in infants with single ventricle: results of a multicenter randomized trial. Circulation 2010; 122(4): 333-40.
[http://dx.doi.org/10.1161/CIRCULATIONAHA.109.927988] [PMID: 20625111]

[86] Thompson LD, McElhinney DB, Culbertson CB, *et al.* Perioperative administration of angiotensin converting enzyme inhibitors decreases the severity and duration of pleural effusions following bidirectional cavopulmonary anastomosis. Cardiol Young 2001; 11(2): 195-200.
[http://dx.doi.org/10.1017/S1047951101000105] [PMID: 11293738]

[87] Lee K-J, Yoo S-J, Holtby H, *et al.* Acute effects of the ACE inhibitor enalaprilat on the pulmonary, cerebral and systemic blood flow and resistance after the bidirectional cavopulmonary connection. Heart 2011; 97(16): 1343-8.
[http://dx.doi.org/10.1136/hrt.2011.225656] [PMID: 21646245]

[88] Packer M, Gheorghiade M, Young JB, *et al.* Withdrawal of digoxin from patients with chronic heart failure treated with angiotensin-converting-enzyme inhibitors. RADIANCE Study. N Engl J Med 1993; 329(1): 1-7.
[http://dx.doi.org/10.1056/NEJM199307013290101] [PMID: 8505940]

[89] Kimball TR, Daniels SR, Meyer RA, *et al.* Effect of digoxin on contractility and symptoms in infants with a large ventricular septal defect. Am J Cardiol 1991; 68(13): 1377-82.
[http://dx.doi.org/10.1016/0002-9149(91)90249-K] [PMID: 1951128]

[90] Seguchi M, Nakazawa M, Momma K. Further evidence suggesting a limited role of digitalis in infants with circulatory congestion secondary to large ventricular septal defect. Am J Cardiol 1999; 83(9): 1408-1411, A8.
[http://dx.doi.org/10.1016/S0002-9149(99)00109-5] [PMID: 10235104]

[91] Gottlieb SS, Fisher ML, Kjekshus J, *et al.* Tolerability of β-blocker initiation and titration in the Metoprolol CR/XL Randomized Intervention Trial in Congestive Heart Failure (MERIT-HF). Circulation 2002; 105(10): 1182-8.
[http://dx.doi.org/10.1161/hc1002.105180] [PMID: 11889011]

[92] Packer M, Fowler MB, Roecker EB, *et al.* Effect of carvedilol on the morbidity of patients with severe chronic heart failure: results of the carvedilol prospective randomized cumulative survival (COPERNICUS) study. Circulation 2002; 106(17): 2194-9.
[http://dx.doi.org/10.1161/01.CIR.0000035653.72855.BF] [PMID: 12390947]

[93] Gheorghiade M, Colucci WS, Swedberg K. Beta-blockers in chronic heart failure. Circulation 2003; 107(12): 1570-5.
[http://dx.doi.org/10.1161/01.CIR.0000065187.80707.18] [PMID: 12668487]

[94] Shaddy RE, Tani LY, Gidding SS, *et al.* Beta-blocker treatment of dilated cardiomyopathy with

congestive heart failure in children: a multi-institutional experience. J Heart Lung Transplant 1999; 18(3): 269-74.
[http://dx.doi.org/10.1016/S1053-2498(98)00030-8] [PMID: 10328154]

[95]   Kalay N, Basar E, Ozdogru I, *et al.* Protective effects of carvedilol against anthracycline-induced cardiomyopathy. J Am Coll Cardiol 2006; 48(11): 2258-62.
[http://dx.doi.org/10.1016/j.jacc.2006.07.052] [PMID: 17161256]

[96]   Schmidt B, Andrew M. Neonatal thrombosis: report of a prospective Canadian and international registry. Pediatrics 1995; 96(5 Pt 1): 939-43.
[PMID: 7478839]

[97]   Baird CW, Zurakowski D, Robinson B, *et al.* Anticoagulation and pediatric extracorporeal membrane oxygenation: impact of activated clotting time and heparin dose on survival. Ann Thorac Surg 2007; 83(3): 912-9.
[http://dx.doi.org/10.1016/j.athoracsur.2006.09.054] [PMID: 17307433]

[98]   Coombs CJ, Richardson PW, Dowling GJ, Johnstone BR, Monagle P, Coombs CJ, *et al.* Brachial artery thrombosis in infants: an algorithm for limb salvage. Plast Reconstr Surg 2006; 117(5): 1481-8.
[http://dx.doi.org/10.1097/01.prs.0000206311.92369.73] [PMID: 16641716]

[99]   Newall F, Johnston L, Ignjatovic V, Summerhayes R, Monagle P. Age-related plasma reference ranges for two heparin-binding proteins--vitronectin and platelet factor 4. Int J Lab Hematol 2009; 31(6): 683-7.
[http://dx.doi.org/10.1111/j.1751-553X.2008.01107.x] [PMID: 19909382]

[100]   Newall F, Savoia H, Campbell J, Monagle P. Anticoagulation clinics for children achieve improved warfarin management. Thromb Res 2004; 114(1): 5-9.
[http://dx.doi.org/10.1016/j.thromres.2004.03.018] [PMID: 15262478]

[101]   Monagle P, Newall F, Campbell J. Anticoagulation in neonates and children: Pitfalls and dilemmas. Blood Rev 2010; 24(4-5): 151-62.
[http://dx.doi.org/10.1016/j.blre.2010.06.003] [PMID: 20663595]

CHAPTER 3

Hypertrophic Cardiomyopathy in Pediatric Population

Sarah Moharem Elgamal*, Shehab M. Anwer and **Mohammad El Tahlawi#**

Bristol Heart Institute, University Hospitals Bristol NHS Trust, Bristol, UK

 # Zagazig University, Egypt

Abstract: Hypertrophic cardiomyopathy (HCM) is an inherited autosomal dominant genetic disease characterised by asymmetrical increased wall thickness of a non-dilated LV chamber. It has a diverse natural history which is attributed to its heterogeneous clinical presentation. HCM could be diagnosed clinically, by ECG changes and definitely by echocardiographic characteristics. Pharmacological therapy has an important role in the management of HCM. Alcohol septal ablation and pacing may be used in certain conditions. Septal myectomy, Morrow procedure, is indicated to reduce persistent gradient and alleviate symptoms refractory to medications.

Keywords: Cardiomyopathy, Congenital Heart Disease, Dual Chamber Pacing, End-Stage Heart Failure, Gene Mutation, Hypertrophy, Myectomy, Morrow, Outflow Obstruction, Septal Ablation, Sudden Cardiac Death.

1. INTRODUCTION

Hypertrophic cardiomyopathy in children is defined as an increased wall thickness of a non-dilated LV chamber by more than two standard deviations, in the absence of an identifiable abnormal loading conditions or systemic disease capable of producing the magnitude of hypertrophy [1]. Since the initial recognition of HCM almost 60 years ago [2, 3], the perception, diagnosis and management of this condition have progressed over the past 2 decades and continue to evolve with the establishment of modern registries, the clinical availability of genetic testing and advances in therapeutic interventions as a result of the dedicated efforts from HCM centers of excellence.

Pediatric onset HCM is similar to adult onset if the disease etiology is sarcomeric. However, a substantial number of syndromes and conditions present with an

---

*** Corresponding author Sarah Moharem Elgamal:** Bristol Heart Institute, University Hospitals Bristol NHS Trust, Bristol, UK; Tel: +4411734226569; E-mail: sarah.elgamal@bristol.ac.uk

Mohammad El Tahlawi (Ed.)
All rights reserved-© 2020 Bentham Science Publishers

HCM phenotype requires a different therapeutic strategy than that used to manage "primary HCM" [4]. In this chapter, the main focus will be on sarcomeric hypertrophic cardiomyopathy with a brief discussion of its differential diagnosis.

2. ETIOLOGY

Our understanding of HCM has evolved since Dr. Donald Teare first described "asymmetrical hypertrophy of the young" in 1958 [2]. HCM presenting in infancy and childhood can be caused due to a wide spectrum of etiologies. Sarcomeric gene mutations are identified in 40-60% of patients presenting with HCM [5 - 8].

HCM is a prototypic single-gene disorder and commonly familial disease. It is inherited in an autosomal dominant mode. It is sporadic in about one-third of cases. The genetic basis of HCM has not been completely clarified [9].

In "primary" HCM at least 450 mutations in 27 sarcomeric and myofilament-related proteins have been identified as disease causing mutations [10 - 13]. These missense, nonsense, or frame shift gene mutations are usually inherited as an autosomal dominant trait. Other modes of transmission include autosomal recessive and de novo mutations. Mutations of the cardiac sarcomere proteins contribute to about 50% of pediatric onset HCM [5, 14]. However, cardiac sarcomere gene mutations were attributed to 11-17% of infantile onset HCM [5, 11, 15]. Sarcomeric and myofilament-related proteins gene causing mutations are listed in Table **1**.

Table 1. Sarcomeric and myofilament-related proteins gene causing mutations.

Gene	Protein	Frequency in HCM Patients
MYH7	β-Myosin heavy chain	25–35%
MYBPC3	Myosin-binding protein C	25-30%
TNNT2	Troponin T	3–5%
TNNI3	Troponin I	<5%
TPM1	Tropomyosin 1α	<5%
MYL2	Regulatory myosin light chain 2	<5%
MYL3	Essential myosin light chain 3	Rare
ACTC	α-Cardiac actin 1	Rare
TTN	Titin	Rare
TNNC1	Troponin C, slow skeletal and cardiac muscles	Rare
MYH6	α-Myosin heavy chain	Rare
CSRP3	Muscle LIM protein	Rare

(Table 1) cont.....

Gene	Protein	Frequency in HCM Patients
MYLK2	Myosin light chain kinase 2	Rare
LDB3	LIM binding domain 3	Rare
TCAP	telethonin	Rare
VCL	Vinculin/metavinculin	Rare
ACTN2	α-Actinin 2	Rare
PLN	Phospholamban	Rare
MYOZ2	Myozenin 2	Rare
JPH2	Junctophilin 2	Rare

MYBPC3 and MYH7 are the most commonly identified sarcomeric gene mutations, accounting for 80% of all genotype-positive patients [6, 8, 16 - 18].

Myosin heavy chain 7 or β-myosin heavy chain and myosin binding protein C, the 2 major components of the sarcomeres, are encoded by these genes. *MYBPC3 is more liable to* insertion/deletion and frame shift mutations than *MYH7* gene [8, 19, 20]. (*TNNT2, TNNI3,* and *TPM1* account for less than 10% of cases. They encode the thin filament proteins cardiac troponin T, cardiac troponin I, and α-tropomyosin [8]. Other gene mutations have been reported as possible etiology of HCM. They include genes that code for sarcomere and sarcomere-associated proteins as titin (*TTN*), cardiac α-actin (*ACTC*), telethonin *(TCAP)*, myosin light chain 2 (*MYL2*), myosin light chain 3 (*MYL3*), myozenin 2 (*MYOZ2*), and ubiquitin E3 ligase tripartite motif protein 63 (*TRIM63*) [21, 22]. In general, genes responsible for approximately 60% of HCM have been identified. The remainder are responsible for some sporadic cases or HCM occurring in small families [23].

Phenotypic expression of HCM is highly variable, even among family members sharing the same gene mutation [24]. The widespread commercial availability of genetic counseling and testing has allowed the identification of an emerging population of phenonegative genopositive family members before the overt expression of the disease. The identification of these individuals will allow us to better understand the natural history of disease and identify the factors that contribute to disease expression. This could eventually lead to the development of novel therapies that may prevent the manifestation of HCM.

Other several conditions in which primary left ventricular hypertrophy (LVH) constitutes an important pathological feature and clinically resembles HCM are considered as phenocopy HCM. The pathophysiology of hypertrophy in such conditions includes mutations in genes other than those coding for sarcomere proteins [9].

These secondary causes that mimic HCM in a pediatric population include inborn errors of metabolism, mitochondrial disorders, neuromuscular and malformation syndromes [25]. It is important that these causes are identified, as additional medical management will be required. Conditions that mimic HCM (HCM phenocopies) account for less than 10% of hypertrophy in childhood. A list of HCM phenocopies' etiologies, gene affected, mode of inheritance and characteristic extracardiac clinical features is displayed in Table **2**.

Table 2. List of HCM phenocopies' etiologies, gene affected and mode of inheritance and characteristic extracardiac clinical features.

Disease Condition	Gene Affected	Mode of Inheritance	Extracardiac Features
Anderson–Fabry	*GLA*	X-linked	Renal disease, paraesthesia/ neuropathic pain, Ensorineural deafness, corneal opacity, excessive sweating
Danon	*LAMP2*	X-linked	Visual impairment
AMP kinase disease PRKAG2	*PRKAG2*	AD	Muscle pain and stiffness
LEOPARD syndrome	*PTPN11, RAF1, BRAF, and MAP2K1*	AD	Lentigines, ocular hypertelorism, pulmonary stenosis, abnormal genitalia, retarded growth and sensorineural deafness (males often have genital abnormalities).
Noonan	*PTPN11, SOS1, RAF1, and RIT1*	AD	Learning difficulties/ mental retardation, hypertelorism, ptosis, low set ears, and a short, webbed neck, scoliosis and a short stature.
Friedreich's ataxia	*FXN*	AR	Gait disturbance, gradual loss of strength and sensation in the arms and legs; muscle stiffness (spasticity); and impaired speech, hearing, and vision
Pompe	*GAA*	AR	Muscle weakness (myopathy), hypotonia and hepatomegaly.
Cori disease	*AGL*	AR	Muscle weakness and hepatomegaly.
Mitochondrial diseases: Kearns–Sayre MELAS MERRF	Mitochondrial DNA deletions *MT-TL1 MT-TK*	mitochondrial pattern (maternal inheritance)	Learning difficulties/ mental retardation, muscle weakness and visual impairment.

2.1. Genotype-Phenotype Relationship

Patients with HCM are considerably variable in the clinical severity, degree of hypertrophy and risk of SCD [24, 26]. Several genetic variants and epigenetic factors causing the phenotypic variability of HCM through influencing the expression of the phenotype in each patient. The causal mutation constitutes the largest influence on the phenotype. However, many other determinants are still unknown. Phenotypic variability (expressivity), variable penetrance, and pleiotropy (multiple phenotypes associated with a single gene or genetic variants) comprise genotype-phenotype relationship and decrease the predictive value of genetic testing in HCM [27, 28].

3. EPIDEMIOLOGY AND NATURAL HISTORY

Historically, HCM was perceived as a rare condition with a poor prognosis. This misconception was proved wrong by contemporary epidemiological studies that demonstrated HCM has a relatively benign clinical course with longevity similar to that of the general population [29 - 32]. Worldwide, HCM is the most commonly inherited cardiac disease with a prevalence of about 0.2% (1: 500) [33, 34]. The prevalence within a pediatric population is unknown, but registries from different continents have shown the annual incidence of HCM to be about 3-5 per 1 million children [35].

HCM's diverse natural history is attributed to its heterogeneous clinical presentation and its variable penetrance [36]. Children with familial hypertrophic cardiomyopathy present significantly later than those with non-familial hypertrophic cardiomyopathy. The cause for the differences in clinical expression is still elusive, even among family members who share the same disease causing mutations. Possible determining factors include modifier genes and environmental factors [24]. In children and adolescents, growth hormones may also be a contributing factor.

LVOT obstruction, burnt out HCM, atrial fibrillation, stroke and sudden cardiac death are severe clinical features of the disease spectrum that alter the clinical course of HCM if necessary therapeutic measurements are not undertaken [37]. Infants diagnosed with LVH in their first year of life are more likely to have non-sarcomeric mimicking etiology with a poor outcome, while those presenting after the age of 1 year have a mortality rate of 1–1.5% [35, 38]. HCM is the leading cause of sudden cardiac death (SCD) in the young [39]. It is commonly linked to playing competitive sports or vigorous exertion. One study reported the annual incidence of sudden cardiac death of HCM patients' ages 9–13.9 years to be as high as 7.2% [40].

4. DIAGNOSIS

4.1. Clinical Presentation

Children with HCM may present immediately after birth or early infancy to later during childhood and adolescence. An early age of presentation and additional extracardiac features identified during clinical assessment make a diagnosis of HCM phenocopies more likely. Extracardiac features include dysmorphic facial features, retarded growth and skeletal deformities, muscle weakness and hypotonia, ataxia, impaired mental status and hepatomegaly. These features warrant further evaluation by other specialties (genetics, metabolism and neurology) to reach a diagnosis.

HCM may be asymptomatic, only to be discovered by the incidental auscultation of a murmur. In some cases, it is identified during family screening or an abnormal ECG prior to participating in competitive sports.

Symptomatic patients may present with:

Symptoms of congestive heart failure (with preserved systolic function) include:

- Difficulty in feeding for infants and younger children;
- Decreased exercise capacity and exertional dyspnea in older children;
- Paroxysmal nocturnal dyspnea;
- Orthopnea.
- Palpitations due to supraventricular or ventricular arrhythmias.
- Angina due to myocardial supply demand mismatch as a result of structural microvascular abnormalities.
- Dizziness, presyncope or syncope due to arrhythmia or LVOTO.
- Sudden cardiac death is the most devastating and sometimes the only manifestation.

Physical examination may be normal in the patients with hypertrophic non-obstructive cardiomyopathy. The following abnormalities may be detected on examination in patients with hypertrophic obstructive cardiomyopathy:

The arterial pulse may be bifid, in which an initial rapid upstroke is felt due to a sudden increase blood flow from the center ventricular outflow tract to the aorta. Then, a sudden down stroke occurs during mid-systole as a result of the development of the left ventricular outflow tract gradient. This is then followed by a second upstroke. A prominent 'a' wave may be noticed upon examination of the jugular venous pulse in the presence of diminished right ventricular compliance secondary to ventricular septal hypertrophy.

Upon examination of the heart, the apex is usually displaced laterally with a systolic lift (bulge). A systolic thrill may felt at the apex or along the lower left sternal border in mitral regurge and left ventricular obstruction respectively. The first and second heart sounds (S1 and S2) are usually normal in patients with HCM. The intensity of S1 decreases in the presence of mitral regurgitation. S2 maybe paradoxically split in patients with subaortic gradients. A third heart sound (S3) or gallop is common in children with HCM, but is of much less clinical significance than the S3 heard in valvular aortic stenosis or in heart failure patients. A fourth heart sound (S4) is frequently heard due to atrial systole against a stiff left ventricle.

In patients with outflow obstruction, a loud crescendo-decrescendo systolic murmur is heard along the left parasternal border. The intensity of the murmur is directly proportionate to the degree of obstruction in the left ventricular outflow tract. As left ventricular outflow obstruction is dynamic, the murmur may not always be audible (i.e. latent) and its intensity varies from one examination to the other. On dynamic auscultation, maneuvers that decrease the left ventricle's preload, such as standing, Valsalva maneuver and administration of diuretics or nitrates, increase the intensity of the murmur. The murmur also becomes louder with reduced afterload and increase of myocardial contractility.

In HOCM patients, a pansystolic murmur of mitral regurgitation may be heard at the apex and propagating to the left axilla. This occurs during midsystole as a result of suction of the anterior mitral valve leaflet into the obstructed left ventricular outflow. In this scenario, the severity of the mitral regurge may be proportional to the degree of left ventricular outflow obstruction. Similarly changes in the heart's loading conditions can also affect the degree of severity of mitral regurge. If the mitral regurgitation murmur propagates to the left parasternal border, then this is likely due to an associated intrinsic abnormality of the mitral valve apparatus.

4.2. Investigations

4.2.1. Laboratory Blood Tests

No specific laboratory blood tests are required in the workup of "primary" HCM. Genetic testing is recommended and commercially available (discussed later).

4.2.2. Electrocardiogram

Seventy five to 95% of HCM patients show ECG abnormalities [41]. These abnormalities are usually in the form of ST-T wave deviations, increased QRS voltage indicative of left ventricular hypertrophy, axis deviation and abnormal and prominent Q waves mimicking myocardial infarction. Conduction abnormalities may also be observed in the form of PR prolongation or bundle branch block. Arrhythmias as atrial fibrillation/flutter may be noted. Patients with mild hypertrophy may have a normal ECG. Moreover, studies of phenonegative genopositive family members have shown that ECG abnormalities, as early repolarization, can manifest before overt hypertrophy.

The presence of an extremely large QRS voltage (Sokolow score $\geq$50) may be observed in HCM phenocopies. A short PR interval with slurring and slow rise of the initial upstroke of the widened QRS complex (delta wave) has been associated with non-sarcomeric HCM causing gene mutations as AMP-activated PRKAG2, LAMP2 and GLA.

4.2.3. Chest X-ray

The cardiac silhouette may be increased. Patients presenting with heart failure symptoms may have increased pulmonary vascular markings.

4.2.4. Echocardiography

In children, increased LV wall thickness is defined as wall thickness $\geq$ 2 standard deviations above the mean (Z score $\geq$ 2) for age, sex, or body size [1]. The basal septum is the usual site of maximum hypertrophy, but other segments, as the posterior and apical, may also be affected. M-mode imaging allows the identification of asymmetric hypertrophy of the septal to the posterior wall, a ratio of $\geq$ 1.5 [42]. In 1985, Maron proposed the following classification to describe the distribution of hypertrophy by 2D echocardiography parasternal short axis view:

Type I: Confined to anterior segment of ventricular septum.
Type II: Involving anterior and posterior septum.
Type III: Substantial portions of both septum and free wall.
Type IV: Regions other than the basal and anterior septum [43].

If the distribution of hypertrophy is concentric, other cardiac conditions as well as infiltrative cardiomyopathy should be excluded.

In the presence of obstruction, premature closure of the aortic valve with mid-systolic notching will be noted. If an early systolic notch is observed, the examiner should exclude the presence of a subaortic membrane (Fig. **1**). Left atrial diameter may be increased in the presence of LVOT obstruction, diastolic dysfunction and/or mitral regurge. An increased diameter is associated with a higher incidence of atrial fibrillation, heart failure development and death [44]. The presence and grade of systolic anterior motion (SAM) of the anterior mitral valve leaflet has also been used to demonstrate the presence and degree of LVOT obstruction [45] Fig. (**2**).

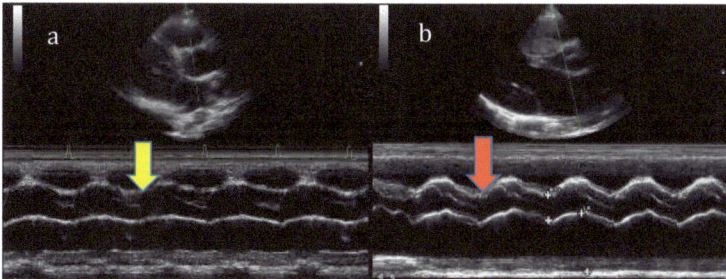

Fig. (1). The upper left panel (a) is an M-mode echocardiogram of an HOCM patient shows premature closure of the aortic valve with mid-systolic notching (yellow arrow). The upper right panel (b) is an M-M mode echocardiogram of a patient with a subaortic membrane. It shows premature closure of the aortic valve with mid-systolic notching (yellow arrow).

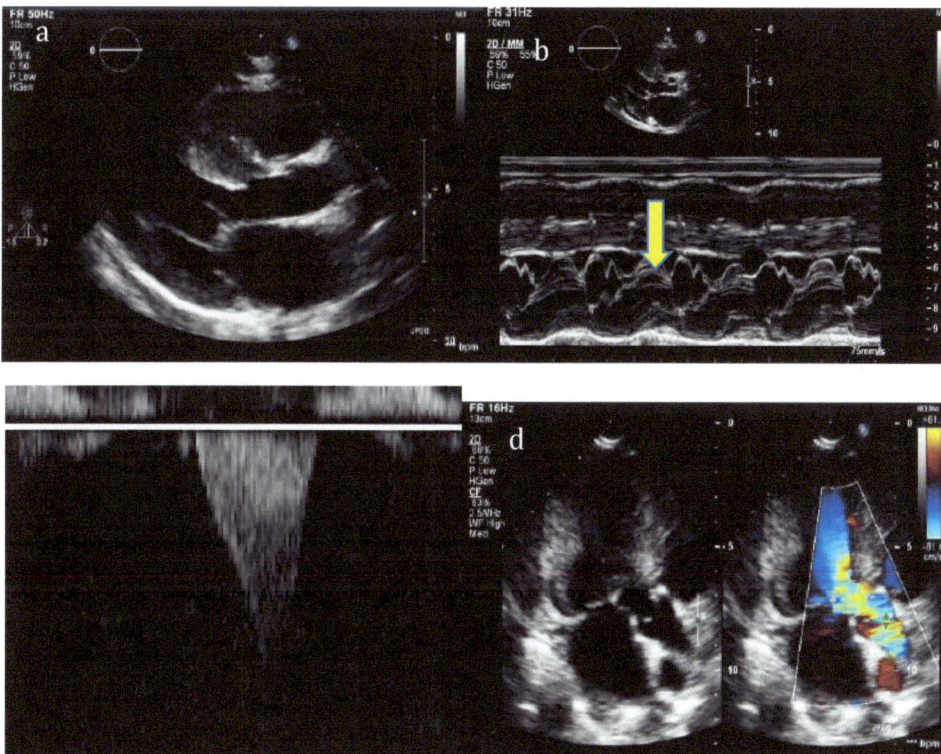

Fig. (2). The upper left panel (a) is 2D echocardiogram parasternal long axis view of a patient with septal hypertrophy and systolic anterior motion of the mitral leaflet [SAM (arrow)]. The upper right panel b) is an M-mode echocardiogram of a patient with septal hypertrophy and systolic anterior motion of the mitral leaflet [SAM (arrow)]. The lower left panel (c) is an continuous wave Doppler echocardiogram taken at the LVOT of a patient with HOCM. The lower right panel (d) is a 2D echocardiogram apical 3 chamber view of a patient with LVOTO. As a result of the obstruction, turbulence by color flow is seen.

The assessment of systolic function by ejection fraction is usually normal or even "supernormal". Patients with HCM typically have a small LV cavity and the LV systolic dimensions may be less than normal. Pulse wave Doppler mitral inflow patterns, tissue Doppler tracings and left atrial volume measurement are used to assess LV diastolic function. Impaired LV diastolic function is seen with decreased compliance of the stiff left ventricle [46]. Color flow and Doppler echocardiography are used to identify the presence of obstruction as this has important implications for the patient's management.

4.2.5. Holter Honitoring

Holter monitoring allows the identification of atrial and ventricular arrhythmias. On initial assessment, recent guidelines recommended 48 hour monitoring followed by serial reassessment annually (more frequent monitoring maybe warranted in the presence of left atrial dilatation) [47].

4.2.6. Exercise Testing

Exercise-related hypotension is an established risk factor of SCD in patients younger than 40 years of age [47]. A maximum symptom-limited treadmill exercise test of medications using a standard Bruce protocol or modified Bruce is used to assess the blood pressure response. Exercise-related hypotension is defined as a failure of blood pressure to rise by at least 20 mm Hg from rest to peak exercise or a fall of >20 mm Hg from peak pressure [48]. A symptom-limited treadmill exercise test is also used to provoke a latent LVOTO gradient and detect the presence/ increase severity of mitral regurge with exercise.

4.2.7. Cardiac MRI

In most HCM patients, transthoracic echocardiography is sufficient to identify LV hypertrophy, its pattern of distribution, assess the presence and measure the LVOTO gradient. However, this may not always be achieved in patients with poor acoustic windows or if some of the LV segments cannot be visualized [9, 49]. This can be overcome by the use of cardiac magnetic resonance imaging (CMR). But CMR should not be restricted to just this group of patients. CMR's capability to accurately evaluate anatomy, quantitate chamber size and function, flow quantification, and characterize tissue [50], making its use a routine of the comprehensive initial assessment and follow up of HCM in many centers. Its high spatial and temporal resolution and lack of ionizing radiation make it an attractive complimentary tool in the pediatric population. However, the exam time may be lengthy, young and uncooperative children may require anesthesia and contrast administration is needed for tissue characterization.

This complementary imaging modality provides detailed information of the variable phenotypic expression of HCM. It can reliably visualize the site, pattern and extent of the hypertrophy and accurately measure the wall thickness, even in patients with apical and lateral hypertrophy (Fig. **3**) [51]. It also depicts LV aneurysms and thrombi that may be missed by echocardiography [51 - 53]. Although echocardiography is superior in the assessment of LVOTO, CMR velocity encoded phase sequences can be used to measure the peak velocity of blood flow in the outflow track. The pattern of fibrosis in HCM is diverse in location and pattern, but typically focal midwall enhancement is seen at the RV insertion points [54]. The distribution of hypertrophy and delayed enhancement may help in differentiating HCM from its phenocopies. CMR is also popular in the assessment and follow up of phenonegative genopositive family members. It can reliably detect subtle morphological abnormalities, such as myocardial crypts [55, 56], elongated mitral valve leaflets [57] and papillary muscle abnormalities. Serial assessment may accurately detect an increased LV mass in these individuals prior to overt hypertrophy. The role of cardiac MRI in HCM and its phenocopies is discussed further in Chapter _6_: The Role of Cardiac Imaging in Heart Failure.

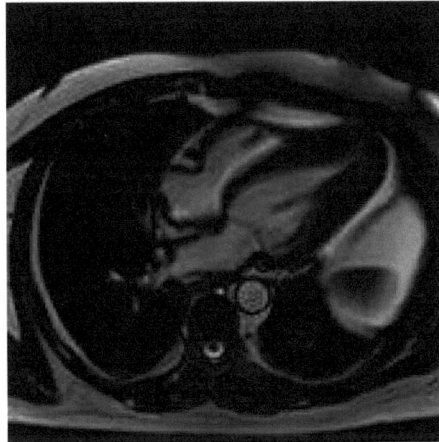

Fig. (3). A cardiac MRI SSFP image 4 chamber orientation of a patient with apical HCM.

4.2.8. Genetic Counseling and Testing

Genetic counseling and testing should be available to all patients and their families to discuss their genetic status, mode and risks of inheritance and to make informed decisions about future pregnancies [58]. Genetic testing is done in accordance to the child's best interests [47, 59]. The most recent guidelines encouraged genetic testing for children 10 years and older should be involved in the decision making for testing and the decision of testing younger children at the parents' discretion [47]. When the clinical diagnosis is unclear, genetic testing is capable of differentiating sarcomeric HCM from phenocopies. This is of utmost importance, as both conditions have a different mode of inheritance, natural history, management and outcome.

HCM is the most common inherited heart disease with an autosomal dominant Mendelian pattern [60 - 62]. Offsprings of the proband carry a 50% risk of transmission [8]. Autosomal recessive and denovo mutations are less common modes of transmission [60 - 62]. Clinical screening and genetic counseling and testing of both parents as well as construction of a three- to four-generation family pedigree help to identify the genetic origin and mode of transmission of the disease. Family pedigrees also assist in the identification of other family members at risk of disease development [47]. Modes of transmissions and pedigrees are illustrated in Fig. (**4a**). A family history of HCM, SCD (and the availability of autopsy reports), heart failure of unknown etiology, heart transplant, implantation of a pacemaker or defibrillator and the presence of extracardiac features should be solicited by a trained healthcare professional [47].

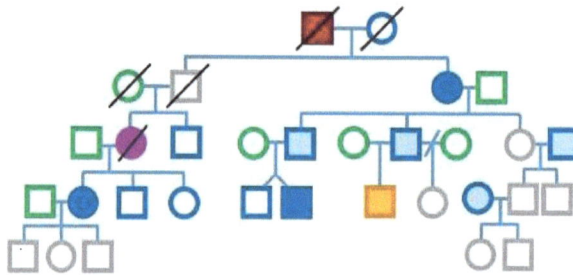

Fig. (4a). Autosomal Dominant Mode of Transmission: The proband will either have inherited the disease causing mutation from either one of his parents. The offsprings of the proband will carry a 50% risk of transmission.

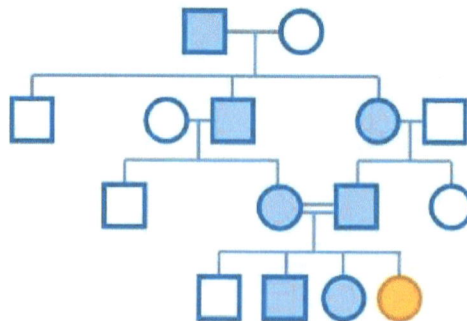

Fig. (4b). Autosomal Reccessive Mode of Transmission: The proband will have inherited the disease causing mutation from both of his/her parents. The proband is homozygous for this condition.

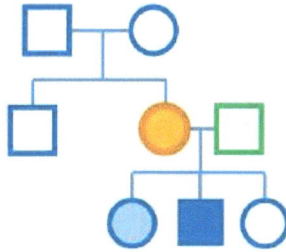

Fig. 4c. Denovo Mode of Transmission: The proband will have not inherited the disease causing mutation from his/her parents, but rather as a result of a **mutation** in a germ cell of one of the parents or the fertilized egg itself. Even though the proband didn't inherit this mutation, the risk of transmission to the next generation is 50% with each offspring.

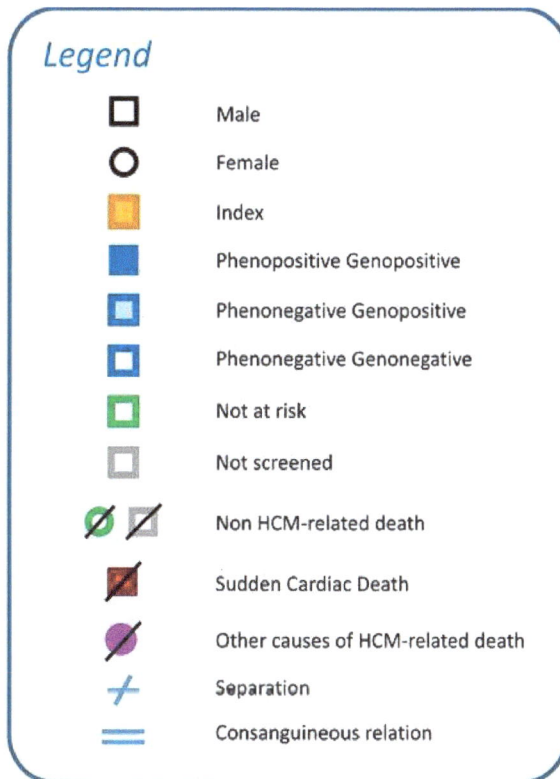

When the molecular diagnosis is confirmed and a single pathogenic (or likely pathogenic) mutation is identified, the clinical diagnosis, management and prognosis are unaffected [63, 64]. The detection of a mutation allows screening of first-degree family members for the same mutation, as they have a 50% risk of carrying the gene. Conversely, double or compound heterozygote mutations have been associated with a severe clinical phenotype that manifests earlier in life [65].

This suggests a gene dose effect on the severity of phenotypic expression. If the genetic test results are negative for a mutation, or if the pathogenicity of the mutation detected is unknown [i.e., variant of unknown significance (VUS)], then this strategy cannot be applied to determine whether the proband's relatives are genetically affected. In patients with VUS mutation(s), family cosegregation studies are encouraged to clarify the pathogenicity of mutation(s). If family members are diagnosed with HCM and share the same VUS mutation, this increases the likelihood that this mutation is pathogenic.

In scenarios where a mutation could not be identified (a negative test) or if genetic testing was not carried out, clinical screening is recommended for all first-degree family members. Clinical screening comprises the assessment of symptoms and signs of HCM, ECG and echocardiogram. As the penetrance and expression of the gene is heterogeneous and cannot be predicted, family members with a normal echocardiogram that are either genopositive or have an unknown genetic status, reassessment is recommended every 5 years until the age of 50 years. In younger family members aged 12-18 years, close follow up is recommended every 12- to 18-month, until full physical maturity is reached [47].

4.2.9. HCM Phenocopies

The pathophysiology, natural history and outcome of HCM phenocopies are unlike that of HCM. Genetic testing and confirmation of the molecular diagnosis has strong impact on these patients' management strategy, thus altering their clinical course and prognosis. For example, genetic testing is essential for diagnosis of Pompe, a glycogen storage disease of very poor prognosis without early identification and enzyme replacement therapy. The confirmation of a LAMP2 mutation is also crucial for diagnosis of Danon's disease, which management's strategy usually necessitates heart transplantation.

5. RISK STRATIFICATION OF SCD

SCD risk assessment is a vital part of the clinical evaluation in young HCM patients. This is recommended during initial assessment and is to be repeated every 1–2 years or whenever there is a change in clinical status [30]. Risk stratification comprises clinical and family history, 48-hour ambulatory ECG, TTE (or CMR in the case of poor echo windows) and a symptom-limited exercise test [66, 67].

Clinical features associated with increased risk of SCD are:

a. **Age:** Ages of 10-35 years are associated with increased risk of SCD.
b. **Non-Sustained Ventricular Tachycardia:** Defined as ≥3 consecutive

ventricular beats at ≥120 BPM lasting <30 seconds ambulatory Holter monitoring and is an independent predictor of SCD.

c. **Family History of Premature Sudden Death:** A positive family history of HCM is defined as clinically significant when one or more family members less than the age of 40 years have died suddenly or when a first degree relative with HCM dies suddenly at any age.

d. **Unexplained Syncope:** Particularly in young patients who experience an episode(s) within 6 months of diagnosis.

e. **LV Thickness:** of ≥30 mm or a Z-score ≥6 measured by TTE (or Cardiac MRI in poorly echogenic patients or when there is an atypical distribution of hypertrophy).

f. **Abnormal Exercise Blood Pressure:** Attenuated response or hypotension defined as at a least 20 mm Hg from rest to peak exercise or a fall of >20 mm Hg from peak pressure. It is associated with a higher risk of SCD in young patients [47, 54, 66].

For primary prevention, implantation of an ICD should be considered in children who have two or more major risk factors [47]. To simplify matters, O'Mahony *et al.* developed and validated a HCM Risk-SCD formula to identify the 5-year risk of SCD of HCM patients [30]. The 2014 ESC HCM guidelines recommended that this formula should be used at the initial evaluation and annual or biannual re-evaluation or whenever there is a change in clinical status. However, HCM Risk-SCD formula was not validated in patients <16 years of age, elite athletes, before/after therapeutic interventions to relieve LVOT obstruction or HCM phenocopies [30]. Thus, it should not be used to risk stratify pediatric HCM.

ICD implantation is indicated for secondary prevention of SCD in children who have:

-Survived prior cardiac arrest due to VT or VF;

-Experienced syncope or hemodynamic compromise due to spontaneous sustained VT causing [47].

6. TREATMENT

6.1. General Recommendations

i. Moderate restriction of physical activity is recommended. HCM patients should not take part in strenuous exercise or competitive sports, even in if the patient is asymptomatic, has minimal hypertrophy, no evidence of obstruction, receives medical treatment or has undergone any intervention [39, 67, 68].

ii. Dehydration, the administration of vasodilators or digitalis should be avoided as they increase the LVOT gradient. Diuretics may be given in the least required dosage to relieve symptoms of congestion.

iii. Rule out HCM phenocopies.
iv. Clinical screening of family members and offering genetic counseling.
v. Serial 12-18 months clinical evaluation in the form of history taking, physical examination, ECG, and 2-dimensional echo studies is recommended for all patients 12 to 18 years of age whether they have manifest HCM or are genopositive phenonegative.
vi. Risk stratification for sudden cardiac death (SCD).

6.2. Pharmacological Therapy

For the past 50 years, pharmacological therapy for HCM remains mostly unchanged. The past and present role of pharmacological therapies is to improve the patients' physical capacity, alleviate symptoms and prevent disease progression. Beta-blockers, verapamil and low dose diuretic agents are pharmacological options for symptoms of heart failure, while beta-blockers are prescribed to relieve LVOTO. The usage of disopyramide is not recommended, as no data is currently available regarding its safety in this population.

Current practices are based on observational series and not prospective randomized clinical trials. The impact of the available pharmacological agents to alter the natural history of HCM is still undetermined. Novel therapies, targeting the further development and prevention of the clinical phenotype, are currently under investigation.

6.3. Beta-Blockers

Beta-blockers are the first line of therapy for HCM patients. Its negative chronotropic and inotropic properties improves diastolic filling time and reduces hypercontractile systolic function, thus improving ventricular compliance and reducing LVOTO [69 - 71]. It also relieves symptoms of angina by increasing perfusion time and reducing extravascular compression [72]. Beta-blockers without intrinsic sympathetic or vasodilator activity, as propanolol, atenolol and metoprolol, are prescribed for HCM. Side effects of beta-blockers are easy fatigability, excess bradycardia, hypotension, and bronchospasm.

6.4. Nondihydropyridine Calcium Channel Blockers

Nondihydropyridine calcium channel blocker, verapamil, is a reasonable substitute when beta-blockers can't be give [47, 73]. It, too, has negative chronotropic and inotropic properties. Its usage is associated a better functional capacity, less symptoms and improved LV diastolic filling in HCM patients [74].

It relieves angina in symptomatic, nonobstructive patients [75]. Yet, it should be used cautiously in LVOTO as its vasodilating properties may induce hypotension, hence provoke or increase the gradient and precipitate pulmonary edema. Its use in "burned out" HCM will lead to decompensation of the patient [66]. Dihydropyridine calcium-channel blockers are not recommended in HCM patients.

6.5. Antiarrhythmics

Despite its side effects, amiodarone is the most commonly used antiarrhythmic drug, as it is the safest in structural heart disease [76]. This class III antiarrhythmic agent is used to maintain sinus rhythm in patients with previous episodes of AF prevents potentially life-threatening ventricular arrhythmias and decrease the need of ICD shock discharge.10 The use of digitalis is restricted to control the rate of rapid AF in decompensated patients and/or those with adverse hemodynamic effects.

As previously discussed, ICDS are implanted for secondary prevention of SCD. For primary prevention, the risk-benefit of ICD implantation should be weighed. It is indicated if the patient has 2 or more risk factors of SCD or for secondary prevention. The inappropriate shocks discharged by the ICDs may lead to a poorer quality of life, anxiety and depression. The use of beta-blockers and/or amiodarone is recommended in patients with an ICD to decrease recurrent appropriate shocks.

6.6. Interventions to Relieve LVOTO

6.6.1. Myectomy

Septal myectomy, Morrow procedure, is indicated to reduce persistent LVOTO gradient ($\geq$ 50 mmHg) and alleviate symptoms refractory to medications [66, 77]. By a transaortic incision, relief of obstruction and widening of the LVOT is done through excision of the hypertrophied, basal interventricular septum (IVS) till the site of maximum impact of the mitral valve leaflet with the septum (Fig. **5**) [77]. An extended septal myectomy is another technique guided by pre-operative imaging of the depth, width and length of muscle hypertrophy [78]. The left and right fibrous trigones are then explored and mobilized by removing the fibrous tissue from the angles of the trigones, thus restoring the normal mobility of the subaortic curtain [79]. Anterior displacement of the papillary muscles or their attachment to the lateral LV wall is corrected by mobilization or thinning of the papillary muscles from the free wall of the LV and excision of the restricted abnormal chords [78, 80].

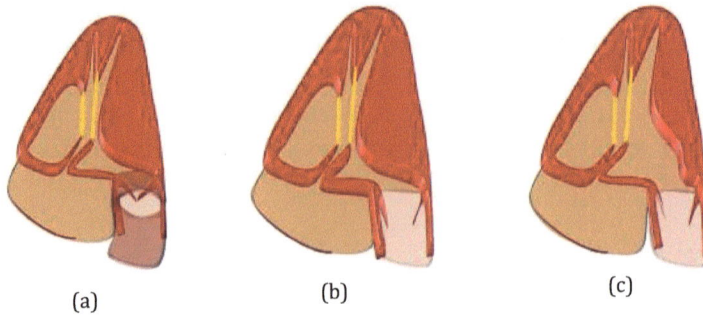

(a)   (b)   (c)

Fig. (5). The steps of the myectomy procedure are illustrated in the cross section images of the heart above. The Marrow procedure starts with median thoracotomy, followed by cannulation of main vessels to go onto cardiopulmonary bypass. After cardioplegia, a transverse incision of the aorta (a) is made to access the LVOT and basal segment of the interventricular septum (IVS) through the aortic valve (b). A small amount of muscle ($\approx$ 5gm) is excised from the hypertrophied IVS extending to the site of maximum impact of the anterior mitral leaflet with the septum (SAM). This widens the LVOT allowing blood to flow normally (c).

Myectomy has a high success rate with substantial improvement of intraventricular flow and symptoms in about 90% of patients [81 - 84]. In experienced centers, the mortality rate is low, ranging from 0% to 5% [85, 86].

Pediatric population results are similar to that of an adult population [87, 88]. But, the recurrence rate is more frequent in pediatric populations in comparison to the adults (2%) [89].

Complications of septal myectomy include:

Left bundle branch block.
Complete heart block requiring permanent pacing in patients with preoperative right bundle branch block or increase QRS duration.
-Ventricular septal defect due to over resection of the IVS (estimated risk of 2%).
Minimal aortic valve injury due to the trans-valvular access. Valve replacement is rarely required.

6.6.2. Dual-Chamber Pacing

In 1995, Dual-chamber pacing (DCP) was used to reduce LVOTO. It was proposed that by asynchronous ventricular pacing, the RV would be stimulated to contract first, thus pulling the interventricular septum in the anterior direction, away from the impact of systolic motion of the anterior leaflet, hence decreasing blood flow turbulence and gradient across the outflow tract [90, 91]. This procedure is not popular nowadays. It is usually restricted for adult patients who can't undergo the other LVOTO relieving procedures or if the patient has another indication for pacing [92].

6.6.3. Alcohol Septal Ablation

This technique is not recommended for the pediatric population as these young patients have small septal artery branches making the procedure technically difficult. Its use is also discouraged in the pediatric age group as the myocardial infarction produced by the procedure may later be a substrate for ventricular arrhythmias [92].

CONSENT FOR PUBLICATION

Not applicable.

CONFLICT OF INTEREST

The authors confirm that this chapter contents have no conflict of interest.

ACKNOWLEDGEMENTS

Declared none.

REFERENCES

[1]   Kampmann C, Wiethoff CM, Wenzel A, *et al.* Normal values of M mode echocardiographic measurements of more than 2000 healthy infants and children in central Europe. Heart 2000; 83(6): 667-72.
[http://dx.doi.org/10.1136/heart.83.6.667] [PMID: 10814626]

[2]   Teare D. Asymmetrical hypertrophy of the heart in young adults. Br Heart J 1958; 20(1): 1-8.
[http://dx.doi.org/10.1136/hrt.20.1.1] [PMID: 13499764]

[3]   Braunwald E, Lambrew CT, Rockoff SD, Ross J Jr, Morrow AG. Idiopathic hypertrophic subaortic stenosis. I. A description of the disease based upon an analysis of 64 patients. Circulation 1964; 30: 4-, 3-119.
[http://dx.doi.org/10.1161/01.CIR.29.5S4.IV-3] [PMID: 14227306]

[4]   Maskatia SA. Hypertrophic cardiomyopathy: infants, children, and adolescents. Congenit Heart Dis 2012; 7(1): 84-92.
[http://dx.doi.org/10.1111/j.1747-0803.2011.00613.x] [PMID: 22222117]

[5]   Van Driest SL, Ommen SR, Tajik AJ, Gersh BJ, Ackerman MJ. Yield of genetic testing in hypertrophic cardiomyopathy. Mayo Clin Proc 2005; 80(6): 739-44.
[http://dx.doi.org/10.1016/S0025-6196(11)61527-9] [PMID: 15945527]

[6]   Kassem HSh, Azer RS, Saber-Ayad M, *et al.* Early results of sarcomeric gene screening from the Egyptian National BA-HCM Program. J Cardiovasc Transl Res 2013; 6(1): 65-80.
[http://dx.doi.org/10.1007/s12265-012-9425-0] [PMID: 23233322]

[7]   Lopes LR, Zekavati A, Syrris P, *et al.* Genetic complexity in hypertrophic cardiomyopathy revealed by high-throughput sequencing. J Med Genet 2013; 50(4): 228-39.
[http://dx.doi.org/10.1136/jmedgenet-2012-101270] [PMID: 23396983]

[8]   Richard P, Charron P, Carrier L, *et al.* Hypertrophic cardiomyopathy: distribution of disease genes, spectrum of mutations, and implications for a molecular diagnosis strategy. Circulation 2003; 107(17): 2227-32.
[http://dx.doi.org/10.1161/01.CIR.0000066323.15244.54] [PMID: 12707239]

[9] Marian AJ, van Rooij E, Roberts R. Genetics and Genomics of Single-Gene Cardiovascular Diseases: Common Hereditary Cardiomyopathies as Prototypes of Single-Gene Disorders. J Am Coll Cardiol 2016; 68(25): 2831-49.
[http://dx.doi.org/10.1016/j.jacc.2016.09.968] [PMID: 28007145]

[10] Seidman JG, Seidman C. The genetic basis for cardiomyopathy: from mutation identification to mechanistic paradigms. Cell 2001; 104(4): 557-67.
[http://dx.doi.org/10.1016/S0092-8674(01)00242-2] [PMID: 11239412]

[11] Keren A, Syrris P, McKenna WJ. Hypertrophic cardiomyopathy: the genetic determinants of clinical disease expression. Nat Clin Pract Cardiovasc Med 2008; 5(3): 158-68.
[http://dx.doi.org/10.1038/ncpcardio1110] [PMID: 18227814]

[12] Maskatia SA. Hypertrophic cardiomyopathy: infants, children, and adolescents. Congenit Heart Dis 2012; 7(1): 84-92.
[http://dx.doi.org/10.1111/j.1747-0803.2011.00613.x] [PMID: 22222117]

[13] Tariq M, Ware SM. Importance of genetic evaluation and testing in pediatric cardiomyopathy. World J Cardiol 2014; 6(11): 1156-65.
[http://dx.doi.org/10.4330/wjc.v6.i11.1156] [PMID: 25429328]

[14] Kaski JP, Syrris P, Esteban MT, *et al.* Prevalence of sarcomere protein gene mutations in preadolescent children with hypertrophic cardiomyopathy. Circ Cardiovasc Genet 2009; 2(5): 436-41.
[http://dx.doi.org/10.1161/CIRCGENETICS.108.821314] [PMID: 20031618]

[15] Kindel SJ, Miller EM, Gupta R, *et al.* Pediatric cardiomyopathy: importance of genetic and metabolic evaluation. J Card Fail 2012; 18(5): 396-403.
[http://dx.doi.org/10.1016/j.cardfail.2012.01.017] [PMID: 22555271]

[16] Girolami F, Olivotto I, Passerini I, *et al.* A molecular screening strategy based on beta-myosin heavy chain, cardiac myosin binding protein C and troponin T genes in Italian patients with hypertrophic cardiomyopathy. J Cardiovasc Med (Hagerstown) 2006; 7(8): 601-7.
[http://dx.doi.org/10.2459/01.JCM.0000237908.26377.d6] [PMID: 16858239]

[17] Rodríguez-García MI, Monserrat L, Ortiz M, *et al.* Screening mutations in myosin binding protein C3 gene in a cohort of patients with Hypertrophic Cardiomyopathy. BMC Med Genet 2010; 11: 67.
[http://dx.doi.org/10.1186/1471-2350-11-67] [PMID: 20433692]

[18] Curila K, Benesova L, Penicka M, *et al.* Spectrum and clinical manifestations of mutations in genes responsible for hypertrophic cardiomyopathy. Acta Cardiol 2012; 67(1): 23-9.
[http://dx.doi.org/10.1080/AC.67.1.2146562] [PMID: 22455086]

[19] Marian AJ, Yu QT, Mares A Jr, Hill R, Roberts R, Perryman MB. Detection of a new mutation in the beta-myosin heavy chain gene in an individual with hypertrophic cardiomyopathy. J Clin Invest. American Society for Clinical Investigation 1992; 1(90): 2156-65.
[http://dx.doi.org/10.1172/JCI116101]

[20] Erdmann J, Daehmlow S, Wischke S, Senyuva M, Werner U, Raible J, *et al.* Mutation spectrum in a large cohort of unrelated consecutive patients with hypertrophic cardiomyopathy 2003.
[http://dx.doi.org/10.1034/j.1399-0004.2003.00151.x]

[21] Marian AJ. Hypertrophic cardiomyopathy: from genetics to treatment. Eur J Clin Invest 2010; 40(4): 360-9.
[http://dx.doi.org/10.1111/j.1365-2362.2010.02268.x] [PMID: 20503496]

[22] Ho CY, Charron P, Richard P, Girolami F, Van Spaendonck-Zwarts KY, Pinto Y. Genetic advances in sarcomeric cardiomyopathies: state of the art. Cardiovasc Res 2015; 105(4): 397-408.
[http://dx.doi.org/10.1093/cvr/cvv025] [PMID: 25634555]

[23] Marian AJ. The case of "missing causal genes" and the practice of medicine: a Sherlock Holmes approach of deductive reasoning. Circ Res 2016; 119(1): 21-4.
[http://dx.doi.org/10.1161/CIRCRESAHA.116.308830] [PMID: 27340268]

[24]   Marian AJ. On genetic and phenotypic variability of hypertrophic cardiomyopathy: nature *versus* nurture. J Am Coll Cardiol 2001; 38(2): 331-4.
[http://dx.doi.org/10.1016/S0735-1097(01)01389-4] [PMID: 11499720]

[25]   Morita H, Rehm HL, Menesses A, *et al.* Shared genetic causes of cardiac hypertrophy in children and adults. N Engl J Med 2008; 358(18): 1899-908.
[http://dx.doi.org/10.1056/NEJMoa075463] [PMID: 18403758]

[26]   Lopes LR, Rahman MS, Elliott PM. A systematic review and meta-analysis of genotype-phenotype associations in patients with hypertrophic cardiomyopathy caused by sarcomeric protein mutations. Heart 2013; 99(24): 1800-11.
[http://dx.doi.org/10.1136/heartjnl-2013-303939] [PMID: 23674365]

[27]   Daw EW, Lu Y, Marian AJ, Shete S. Identifying modifier loci in existing genome scan data. Ann Hum Genet 2008; 72(Pt 5): 670-5.
[http://dx.doi.org/10.1111/j.1469-1809.2008.00449.x] [PMID: 18494837]

[28]   Christodoulou DC, Wakimoto H, Onoue K, *et al.* 5'RNA-Seq identifies Fhl1 as a genetic modifier in cardiomyopathy. J Clin Invest 2014; 124(3): 1364-70. [Internet].
[http://dx.doi.org/10.1172/JCI70108] [PMID: 24509080]

[29]   Maron BJ, Rowin EJ, Casey SA, *et al.* Hypertrophic Cardiomyopathy in Adulthood Associated With Low Cardiovascular Mortality With Contemporary Management Strategies. J Am Coll Cardiol 2015; 65(18): 1915-28.
[http://dx.doi.org/10.1016/j.jacc.2015.02.061] [PMID: 25953744]

[30]   O'Mahony C, Jichi F, Pavlou M, *et al.* A novel clinical risk prediction model for sudden cardiac death in hypertrophic cardiomyopathy (HCM risk-SCD). Eur Heart J 2014; 35(30): 2010-20.
[http://dx.doi.org/10.1093/eurheartj/eht439] [PMID: 24126876]

[31]   Elliott PM, Poloniecki J, Dickie S, *et al.* Sudden death in hypertrophic cardiomyopathy: identification of high risk patients. J Am Coll Cardiol 2000; 36(7): 2212-8.
[http://dx.doi.org/10.1016/S0735-1097(00)01003-2] [PMID: 11127463]

[32]   Maron BJ, Olivotto I, Spirito P, *et al.* Epidemiology of hypertrophic cardiomyopathy-related death: revisited in a large non-referral-based patient population. Circulation 2000; 102(8): 858-64.
[http://dx.doi.org/10.1161/01.CIR.102.8.858] [PMID: 10952953]

[33]   Maron BJ, Gardin JM, Flack JM, Gidding SS, Kurosaki TT, Bild DE. Prevalence of hypertrophic cardiomyopathy in a general population of young adults. Echocardiographic analysis of 4111 subjects in the CARDIA Study. Coronary Artery Risk Development in (Young) Adults. Circulation 1995; 92(4): 785-9.
[http://dx.doi.org/10.1161/01.CIR.92.4.785] [PMID: 7641357]

[34]   Maron BJ. Hypertrophic cardiomyopathy: an important global disease. Am J Med 2004; 116(1): 63-5.
[http://dx.doi.org/10.1016/j.amjmed.2003.10.012] [PMID: 14706671]

[35]   Nugent AW, Daubeney PEF, Chondros P, *et al.* Clinical features and outcomes of childhood hypertrophic cardiomyopathy: results from a national population-based study. Circulation 2005; 112(9): 1332-8.
[http://dx.doi.org/10.1161/CIRCULATIONAHA.104.530303] [PMID: 16116056]

[36]   Baxi AJ, Restrepo CS, Vargas D, Marmol-Velez A, Ocazionez D, Murillo H. Hypertrophic Cardiomyopathy from A to Z: Genetics, Pathophysiology, Imaging, and Management. Radiographics 2016; 36(2): 335-54.
[http://dx.doi.org/10.1148/rg.2016150137] [PMID: 26963450]

[37]   Chapter 2. Natural History of Untreated Hypertrophic Cardiomyopathy. Li Q, Williams L, and Rakowski H. S.S. Naidu (ed.), Hypertrophic Cardiomyopathy: Foreword by Bernard Gersh and Historical Context by Eugene Braunwald, 9 DOI 10.1007/978-1-4471-4956-9_2, © Springer-Verlag London 2015 page 9-22

[38]   Colan SD, Lipshultz SE, Lowe AM, *et al.* Epidemiology and cause-specific outcome of hypertrophic cardiomyopathy in children: findings from the Pediatric Cardiomyopathy Registry. Circulation 2007; 115(6): 773-81.
[http://dx.doi.org/10.1161/CIRCULATIONAHA.106.621185] [PMID: 17261650]

[39]   Maron BJ, Doerer JJ, Haas TS, Tierney DM, Mueller FO. Sudden deaths in young competitive athletes: analysis of 1866 deaths in the United States, 1980-2006. Circulation 2009; 119(8): 1085-92.
[http://dx.doi.org/10.1161/CIRCULATIONAHA.108.804617] [PMID: 19221222]

[40]   Ostman-Smith I, Wettrell G, Keeton B, *et al.* Age- and gender-specific mortality rates in childhood hypertrophic cardiomyopathy. Eur Heart J 2008; 29(9): 1160-7.
[http://dx.doi.org/10.1093/eurheartj/ehn122] [PMID: 18385119]

[41]   Maron BJ. The electrocardiogram as a diagnostic tool for hypertrophic cardiomyopathy: revisited. Ann Noninvasive Electrocardiol 2001; 6(4): 277-9. [editorial].
[http://dx.doi.org/10.1111/j.1542-474X.2001.tb00118.x] [PMID: 11686906]

[42]   Losi MA, Nistri S, Galderisi M, *et al.* Echocardiography in patients with hypertrophic cardiomyopathy: usefulness of old and new techniques in the diagnosis and pathophysiological assessment. Cardiovasc Ultrasound 2010; 8: 7.
[http://dx.doi.org/10.1186/1476-7120-8-7] [PMID: 20236538]

[43]   Maron BJ. Asymmetry in hypertrophic cardiomyopathy: the septal to free wall thickness ratio revisited. Am J Cardiol 1985; 55(6): 835-8. [editorial].
[http://dx.doi.org/10.1016/0002-9149(85)90166-3] [PMID: 3156484]

[44]   Nistri S, Olivotto I, Betocchi S, *et al.* Prognostic significance of left atrial size in patients with hypertrophic cardiomyopathy (from the Italian Registry for Hypertrophic Cardiomyopathy). Am J Cardiol 2006; 98(7): 960-5.
[http://dx.doi.org/10.1016/j.amjcard.2006.05.013] [PMID: 16996883]

[45]   Pollick C, Rakowski H, Wigle ED. Muscular subaortic stenosis: the quantitative relationship between systolic anterior motion and the pressure gradient. Circulation 1984; 69(1): 43-9.
[http://dx.doi.org/10.1161/01.CIR.69.1.43] [PMID: 6537786]

[46]   Nagueh SF, Lakkis NM, Middleton KJ, Spencer WH III, Zoghbi WA, Quiñones MA. Doppler estimation of left ventricular filling pressures in patients with hypertrophic cardiomyopathy. Circulation 1999; 99(2): 254-61.
[http://dx.doi.org/10.1161/01.CIR.99.2.254] [PMID: 9892592]

[47]   Force m, Elliott PM, Anastasakis A, Borger MA, *et al.* 2014 ESC Guidelines on diagnosis and management of hypertrophic cardiomyopathy: the Task Force for the Diagnosis and Management of Hypertrophic Cardiomyopathy of the European Society of Cardiology (ESC). Eur Heart J 2014; 35: 2733-79.

[48]   Sadoul N, Prasad K, Elliott PM, Bannerjee S, Frenneaux MP, McKenna WJ. Prospective prognostic assessment of blood pressure response during exercise in patients with hypertrophic cardiomyopathy. Circulation 1997; 96(9): 2987-91.
[http://dx.doi.org/10.1161/01.CIR.96.9.2987] [PMID: 9386166]

[49]   Andrew CY. To; Ashwat Dhillon; Milind Y. Desai. Cardiac Magnetic Resonance in Hypertrophic Cardiomyopathy. J Am Coll Cardiol Img 2011; 4(10): 1123-37.
[http://dx.doi.org/10.1016/j.jcmg.2011.06.022]

[50]   Banka P, Geva T. Advances in pediatric cardiac MRI. Curr Opin Pediatr 2016; 28(5): 575-83.
[http://dx.doi.org/10.1097/MOP.0000000000000400] [PMID: 27428483]

[51]   Maron MS, Finley JJ, Bos JM, *et al.* Prevalence, clinical significance, and natural history of left ventricular apical aneurysms in hypertrophic cardiomyopathy. Circulation 2008; 118(15): 1541-9.
[http://dx.doi.org/10.1161/CIRCULATIONAHA.108.781401] [PMID: 18809796]

[52]   Moon JC, McKenna WJ. The emerging role of cardiovascular magnetic resonance in refining the

diagnosis of hypertrophic cardiomyopathy. Nat Clin Pract Cardiovasc Med 2009; 6(3): 166-7.
[PMID: 19139744]

[53]   Holloway CJ, Betts TR, Neubauer S, Myerson SG. Hypertrophic cardiomyopathy complicated by
       large apical aneurysm and thrombus, presenting as ventricular tachycardia. J Am Coll Cardiol 2010;
       56(23): 1961.
       [http://dx.doi.org/10.1016/j.jacc.2010.01.078] [PMID: 21109122]

[54]   Rudolph A, Abdel-Aty H, Bohl S, *et al.* Noninvasive detection of fibrosis applying contrast-enhanced
       cardiac magnetic resonance in different forms of left ventricular hypertrophy relation to remodeling. J
       Am Coll Cardiol 2009; 53(3): 284-91.
       [http://dx.doi.org/10.1016/j.jacc.2008.08.064] [PMID: 19147047]

[55]   Brouwer WP, Germans T, Head MC. van d V, Heymans MW, Christiaans I,HouwelingAC, Wilde AA,
       van RossumAC. Multiple myocardial crypts on modified long-axis view are a specific finding in pre-
       hypertrophic HCM mutation carriers. Eur Heart J Cardiovasc Imaging 2012; 13: 292-7.
       [http://dx.doi.org/10.1093/ehjci/jes005] [PMID: 22277119]

[56]   Maron MS, Rowin EJ, Lin D, *et al.* Prevalence and clinical profile of myocardial crypts in
       hypertrophic cardiomyopathy. Circ Cardiovasc Imaging 2012; 5(4): 441-7.
       [http://dx.doi.org/10.1161/CIRCIMAGING.112.972760] [PMID: 22563033]

[57]   Maron MS, Olivotto I, Harrigan C, *et al.* Mitral valve abnormalities identified by cardiovascular
       magnetic resonance represent a primary phenotypic expression of hypertrophic cardiomyopathy.
       Circulation 2011; 124(1): 40-7.
       [http://dx.doi.org/10.1161/CIRCULATIONAHA.110.985812] [PMID: 21670234]

[58]   Lee TM, Chung WK. Genetics and Hypertrophic Cardiomyopathy. Curr Pediatr Rep 2016; 4: 35-44.
       [http://dx.doi.org/10.1007/s40124-016-0097-0]

[59]   Ross LF, Saal HM, David KL, Anderson RR. Technical report: Ethical and policy issues in genetic
       testing and screening of children. Genet Med 2013; 15(3): 234-45.
       [http://dx.doi.org/10.1038/gim.2012.176] [PMID: 23429433]

[60]   Seidman CE, Seidman JG. Identifying sarcomere gene mutations in hypertrophic cardiomyopathy: a
       personal history. Circ Res 2011; 108(6): 743-50.
       [http://dx.doi.org/10.1161/CIRCRESAHA.110.223834] [PMID: 21415408]

[61]   Bos JM, Towbin JA, Ackerman MJ. Diagnostic, prognostic, and therapeutic implications of genetic
       testing for hypertrophic cardiomyopathy. J Am Coll Cardiol 2009; 54(3): 201-11.
       [http://dx.doi.org/10.1016/j.jacc.2009.02.075] [PMID: 19589432]

[62]   Ingles J, Sarina T, Yeates L, *et al.* Clinical predictors of genetic testing outcomes in hypertrophic
       cardiomyopathy. Genet Med 2013; 15(12): 972-7.
       [http://dx.doi.org/10.1038/gim.2013.44] [PMID: 23598715]

[63]   Maron BJ, Maron MS, Semsarian C. Genetics of hypertrophic cardiomyopathy after 20 years: clinical
       perspectives. J Am Coll Cardiol 2012; 60(8): 705-15.
       [http://dx.doi.org/10.1016/j.jacc.2012.02.068] [PMID: 22796258]

[64]   Maron BJ, Ommen SR, Semsarian C, *et al.* Hypertrophic cardiomyopathy: present and future, with
       translation into contemporary cardiovascular medicine. J Am Coll Cardiol 2014; 8;64(1): 83-99.

[65]   Ingles J, Doolan A, Chiu C, Seidman J, Seidman C, Semsarian C. Compound and double mutations in
       patients with hypertrophic cardiomyopathy: implications for genetic testing and counselling. J Med
       Genet 2005, 42(10)e59
       [http://dx.doi.org/10.1136/jmg.2005.033886] [PMID: 16199542]

[66]   Gersh BJ, Maron BJ, Bonow RO, *et al.* 2011 ACCF/AHA Guideline for the Diagnosis and Treatment
       of Hypertrophic Cardiomyopathy: a report of the American College of Cardiology
       Foundation/American Heart Association Task Force on Practice Guidelines. Developed in
       collaboration with the American Association for Thoracic Surgery, American Society of

Echocardiography, American Society of Nuclear Cardiology, Heart Failure Society of America, Heart Rhythm Society, Society for Cardiovascular Angiography and Interventions, and Society of Thoracic Surgeons. J Am Coll Cardiol 2011; 13;58(25): e212-60.

[67]   Maron BJ, Maron MS. Hypertrophic cardiomyopathy. Lancet 2013; 381(9862): 242-55.
        [http://dx.doi.org/10.1016/S0140-6736(12)60397-3] [PMID: 22874472]

[68]   Maron BJ, Udelson JE, Bonow RO, *et al.* American Heart Association Electrocardiography and Arrhythmias Committee of Council on Clinical Cardiology, Council on Cardiovascular Disease in Young, Council on Cardiovascular and Stroke Nursing, Council on Functional Genomics and Translational Biology, and American College of Cardiology. Eligibility and Disqualification Recommendations for Competitive Athletes With Cardiovascular Abnormalities: Task Force 3: Hypertrophic Cardiomyopathy, Arrhythmogenic Right Ventricular Cardiomyopathy and Other Cardiomyopathies, and Myocarditis: A Scientific Statement From the American Heart Association and American College of Cardiology. Circulation 2015; 1;132(22): e273-80.

[69]   Sherrid MV, Pearle G, Gunsburg DZ. Mechanism of benefit of negative inotropes in obstructive hypertrophic cardiomyopathy. Circulation 1998; 97(1): 41-7.
        [http://dx.doi.org/10.1161/01.CIR.97.1.41] [PMID: 9443430]

[70]   Flamm MD, Harrison DC, Hancock EW. Muscular subaortic stenosis. Prevention of outflow obstruction with propranolol. Circulation 1968; 38(5): 846-58.
        [http://dx.doi.org/10.1161/01.CIR.38.5.846] [PMID: 4177137]

[71]   Bourmayan C, Razavi A, Fournier C, *et al.* Effect of propranolol on left ventricular relaxation in hypertrophic cardiomyopathy: an echographic study. Am Heart J 1985; 109(6): 1311-6.
        [http://dx.doi.org/10.1016/0002-8703(85)90357-6] [PMID: 4039882]

[72]   Cohen LS, Braunwald E. Amelioration of angina pectoris in idiopathic hypertrophic subaortic stenosis with beta-adrenergic blockade. Circulation 1967; 35(5): 847-51.
        [http://dx.doi.org/10.1161/01.CIR.35.5.847] [PMID: 6067064]

[73]   Spicer RL, Rocchini AP, Crowley DC, Vasiliades J, Rosenthal A. Hemodynamic effects of verapamil in children and adolescents with hypertrophic cardiomyopathy. Circulation 1983; 67(2): 413-20.
        [http://dx.doi.org/10.1161/01.CIR.67.2.413] [PMID: 6681534]

[74]   Bonow RO, Rosing DR, Epstein SE. The acute and chronic effects of verapamil on left ventricular function in patients with hypertrophic cardiomyopathy 1983.
        [http://dx.doi.org/10.1093/eurheartj/4.suppl_F.57]

[75]   Gistri R, Cecchi F, Choudhury L, *et al.* Effect of verapamil on absolute myocardial blood flow in hypertrophic cardiomyopathy. Am J Cardiol 1994; 74(4): 363-8.
        [http://dx.doi.org/10.1016/0002-9149(94)90404-9] [PMID: 8059699]

[76]   Fananapazir L, Leon MB, Bonow RO, Tracy CM, Cannon RO III, Epstein SE. Sudden death during empiric amiodarone therapy in symptomatic hypertrophic cardiomyopathy. Am J Cardiol 1991; 67(2): 169-74.
        [http://dx.doi.org/10.1016/0002-9149(91)90440-V] [PMID: 1987718]

[77]   Morrow AG, Reitz BA, Epstein SE, *et al.* Operative treatment in hypertrophic subaortic stenosis. Techniques, and the results of pre and postoperative assessments in 83 patients. Circulation 1975; 52(1): 88-102.
        [http://dx.doi.org/10.1161/01.CIR.52.1.88] [PMID: 1169134]

[78]   El-Hamamsy I, Lekadir K, Olivotto I, *et al.* Pattern and degree of left ventricular remodeling following a tailored surgical approach for hypertrophic obstructive cardiomyopathy. Glob Cardiol Sci Pract 2012; 3;2012(1): 9.

[79]   Yacoub MH, El-Hamamsy I, Said K, *et al.* The left ventricular outflow in hypertrophic cardiomyopathy: from structure to function. J Cardiovasc Transl Res 2009; 2(4): 510-7.
        [http://dx.doi.org/10.1007/s12265-009-9153-2] [PMID: 20560010]

[80]	Patel P, Dhillon A, Popovic ZB, *et al.* Left Ventricular Outflow Tract Obstruction in Hypertrophic Cardiomyopathy Patients Without Severe Septal Hypertrophy: Implications of Mitral Valve and Papillary Muscle Abnormalities Assessed Using Cardiac Magnetic Resonance and Echocardiography. Circ Cardiovasc Imaging 2015; 8(7)e003132
	[http://dx.doi.org/10.1161/CIRCIMAGING.115.003132] [PMID: 26082555]

[81]	ten Berg JM, Suttorp MJ, Knaepen PJ, Ernst SM, Vermeulen FE, Jaarsma W. Hypertrophic obstructive cardiomyopathy. Initial results and long-term follow-up after Morrow septal myectomy. Circulation 1994; 90(4): 1781-5.
	[http://dx.doi.org/10.1161/01.CIR.90.4.1781] [PMID: 7923662]

[82]	Ommen SR, Maron BJ, Olivotto I, *et al.* Long-term effects of surgical septal myectomy on survival in patients with obstructive hypertrophic cardiomyopathy. J Am Coll Cardiol 2005; 46(3): 470-6.
	[http://dx.doi.org/10.1016/j.jacc.2005.02.090] [PMID: 16053960]

[83]	Woo A, Williams WG, Choi R, *et al.* Clinical and echocardiographic determinants of long-term survival after surgical myectomy in obstructive hypertrophic cardiomyopathy. Circulation 2005; 111(16): 2033-41.
	[http://dx.doi.org/10.1161/01.CIR.0000162460.36735.71] [PMID: 15824202]

[84]	Dearani JA, Ommen SR, Gersh BJ, Schaff HV, Danielson GK. Surgery insight: Septal myectomy for obstructive hypertrophic cardiomyopathy--the Mayo Clinic experience. Nat Clin Pract Cardiovasc Med 2007; 4(9): 503-12.
	[http://dx.doi.org/10.1038/ncpcardio0965] [PMID: 17712363]

[85]	Robbins RC, Stinson EB. Long-term results of left ventricular myotomy and myectomy for obstructive hypertrophic cardiomyopathy. J Thorac Cardiovasc Surg 1996; 111(3): 586-94.
	[http://dx.doi.org/10.1016/S0022-5223(96)70310-0] [PMID: 8601973]

[86]	Heric B, Lytle BW, Miller DP, Rosenkranz ER, Lever HM, Cosgrove DM. Surgical management of hypertrophic obstructive cardiomyopathy. Early and late results. J Thorac Cardiovasc Surg 1995; 110(1): 195-206.
	[http://dx.doi.org/10.1016/S0022-5223(05)80026-1] [PMID: 7609544]

[87]	Minakata K, Dearani JA, O'Leary PW, Danielson GK. Septal myectomy for obstructive hypertrophic cardiomyopathy in pediatric patients: early and late results. Ann Thorac Surg 2005; 80(4): 1424-9.
	[http://dx.doi.org/10.1016/j.athoracsur.2005.03.109] [PMID: 16181882]

[88]	Menon SC, Ackerman MJ, Ommen SR, *et al.* Impact of septal myectomy on left atrial volume and left ventricular diastolic filling patterns: an echocardiographic study of young patients with obstructive hypertrophic cardiomyopathy. J Am Soc Echocardiogr 2008; 21(6): 684-8.
	[http://dx.doi.org/10.1016/j.echo.2007.11.006] [PMID: 18187287]

[89]	Minakata K, Dearani JA, Schaff HV, O'Leary PW, Ommen SR, Danielson GK. Mechanisms for recurrent left ventricular outflow tract obstruction after septal myectomy for obstructive hypertrophic cardiomyopathy. Ann Thorac Surg 2005; 80(3): 851-6.
	[http://dx.doi.org/10.1016/j.athoracsur.2005.03.108] [PMID: 16122442]

[90]	Slade AK, Sadoul N, Shapiro L, *et al.* DDD pacing in hypertrophic cardiomyopathy: a multicentre clinical experience. Heart 1996; 75(1): 44-9.
	[http://dx.doi.org/10.1136/hrt.75.1.44] [PMID: 8624871]

[91]	Nishimura RA, Trusty JM, Hayes DL, *et al.* Dual-chamber pacing for hypertrophic cardiomyopathy: a randomized, double-blind, crossover trial. J Am Coll Cardiol 1997; 29(2): 435-41.
	[http://dx.doi.org/10.1016/S0735-1097(96)00473-1] [PMID: 9015001]

[92]	Colan SD. Hypertrophic cardiomyopathy in childhood. Heart Fail Clin 2010; 6(4): 433-444, vii-iii.
	[http://dx.doi.org/10.1016/j.hfc.2010.05.004] [PMID: 20869644]

CHAPTER 4

Role of Echocardiography in Heart Failure

Ahmed Aljizeeri*, Mouaz H. Al-Mallah and **Ahmed A. Alsaileek**

King Abdulaziz Cardiac Center, King Abdulaziz Medical City-Riyadh, Riyadh, Kingdom of Saudi Arabia

Abstract: Echocardiography remains the cornerstone of the evaluation and management of heart failure despite the availability of other cardiac imaging modalities. It provides adequate and reliable information on diagnosis, therapeutic options and prognosis in every stage of heart failure. It is reliable, reproducible, widely available and cost-effective tool for the evaluation of heart failure. Echo is fundamental in the initiation and adjustment of medication, patient's selection for device therapy and heart transplantation. Furthermore, it is crucial in the follow up and evaluation of response to advanced therapy. Despite the limitation of echo-derived ejection fraction, it is the single most important factor in the enrollment in clinical trials and therefore, clinical decision making in the daily clinical practice. New advances in echo open promising new frontiers in utility of echo in prevention, detection and management of heart failure.

Keywords: Cardiac Mechanics, Cardiac Resynchronization Therapy, Cardiomyopathy, Coronary Artery Disease, Contrast Echocardiography, Diastolic Dysfunction, Ejection Fraction, Fractional Area Change (FAC), Fractional Shortening, Heart Failure, Implantable Cardioverter-Defibrillator, LV Remodeling, Myocardial Performance Index, Myocardial Viability, Noninvasive Hemodynamic, Quinones Equation, Simpson's Rule, Strain and Strain Rate, Stress Echocardiography, Tei Index, Teaccholz Equation, Tricuspid Annular Plane Systolic Excursion (TAPSE), Wall Motion Score Index.

INTRODUCTION

Echocardiography remains the cornerstone of the evaluation and management of heart failure despite the availability of other cardiac imaging modalities. The epidemic of heart failure in the modern era requires a comprehensive, widely available and cost-effective tool that has diagnostic and prognostic values and can provide information about possible etiology. All the major cardiovascular scientific societies emphasize the significant role of echocardiography in the

* **Corresponding author Ahmed Aljizeeri:** King Abdulaziz Cardiac Center, King Abdulaziz Medical City-Riyadh, Riyadh, Kingdom of Saudi Arabia; Tel: +966 11 8011111; Ext: 10485; E-mail: aljizeeri@yahoo.com

Mohammad El Tahlawi (Ed.)
All rights reserved-© 2020 Bentham Science Publishers

evaluation and management of patients with heart failure [1, 2]. This chapter reviews the role and the future application of echocardiography in the management of patients with heart failure.

Contemporary echocardiographic study includes 2 and 3-dimetional echocardiography, M-mode, pulse and continuous Doppler, color flow Doppler and tissue Doppler imaging (Fig. **1**). There are two types of echocardiography (echo); transthoracic echocardiography (TTE) where images are acquired by an ultrasound probe placed on the chest wall of the patient and transesophageal echocardiography (TEE) where images are acquired by an ultrasound probe passing through the esophagus to image the heart from close proximity. Stress echocardiography is another type of echo used to assess the presence of significant coronary artery disease and the hemodynamic significance of valvular abnormalities. Furthermore, the evaluation of cardiac mechanics with strain, strain rate and speckle tracking allows for detection and quantification of early and small changes in cardiac function in addition to better understanding of the pathophysiology of heart failure. Therefore, it helps in early detection and prevention of cardiac pump failure. Thus, echocardiography provides a comprehensive evaluation of cardiac structure and function including cardiac chambers, muscle mass, pericardium and valvular lesions in both early and advanced stages of heart failure [3 - 7].

ECHOCARDIOGRAPHY AND THE DIAGNOSIS OF HEART FAILURE

Assessment of Left Ventricular Systolic Function

LV global systolic function is crucial in the management of almost all cardiac diseases. It has prognostic implications in coronary artery disease, valvular heart disease and is particularly important in the identification and prognostication of patients with heart failure and cardiomyopathy. Left ventricular systolic function is determined by multiple factors including preload, afterload and contractility. Additionally, heart rate and LV geometry contribute to the global function of the LV. Multiple clinical methods are used for evaluation of LV systolic function including ejection fraction, fractional shortening and pressure-volume analysis [8].

Fractional Shortening

Fractional shortening (FS %) is defined as the percentage change in the minor-axis dimension of the heart. It is a linear measurement derived either from the M-mode or 2D echo. Since the circumferential myocardial fiber shortening plays the major role in determining the stroke volume [9], FS% represents a useful measure of LV systolic function. In fact, it was in included in the diagnostic criteria of cardiomyopathy [10]. FS% is considered normal when $\geq$ 25% and is calculated as FS%= $[(LVD_{diastole} - LVD_{systole}) / LVD_{diastole}]$ X 100 [11].

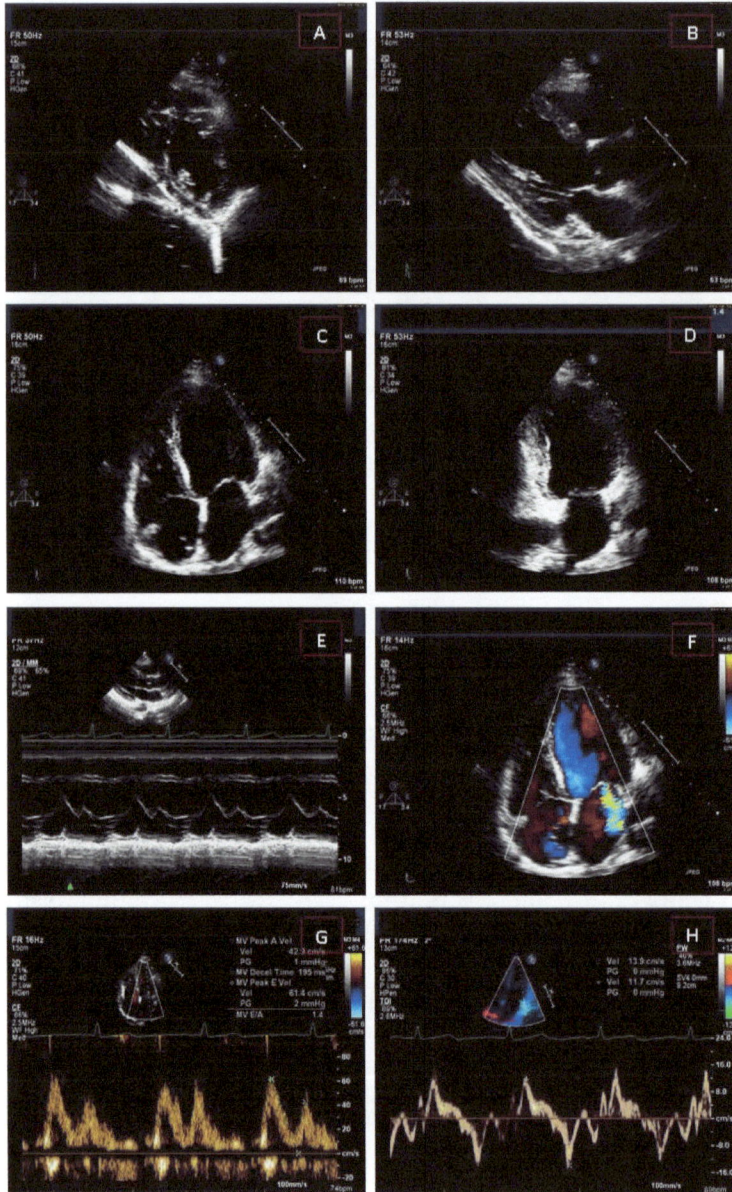

Fig. (1). Components of echocardiographic study: Images A to D show 2-dimentional images of the heart including parasternal short and long axis and apical 2 and 4 chamber views. Image E shows M-Mode, image F shoes color Doppler of mitral regurgitation, image G shows Doppler study of mitral inflow and image H shows tissue Doppler of the lateral mitral annulus.

In normal subjects and clinical conditions where regional wall motion abnormalities are not evident, FS% is very useful and correlates well to left ventricular ejection fraction [12]. However, the presence of regional wall motion abnormalities or ventricular asymmetry can result in inaccuracy of FS% assessment and therefore restricting its use as measure of LV systolic function. In addition, most of the pathological remodeling in the left ventricle occurs in the mid segments and towards the apex further limiting the use of FS% [13]. Thus, its use in routine clinical practice is limited.

LV Ejection Fraction

Left Ventricular Ejection Fraction (LVEF) is the most widely used measure of LV function. It provides a meaningful, measurable and reproducible calculation and synonymously used with left ventricular systolic function. Most of the diagnostic and therapeutic considerations of heart failure are largely based on LVEF.

LVEF is defined as the percentage of blood volume ejected from the LV with each systole and therefore is calculated as LVEF%= (LV stroke volume/ LV end-diastolic volume) X 100 [14]. Hence, assessment of the LVEF is largely dependent on accurate calculation of LV volumes. The estimation of LV volumes is based on theoretical geometric assumption that LV is represented with a mathematical model the dimensions of which can be obtained from the echo studies and therefore the volume can be calculated. The most validated models are biprolate ellipsoid and method of discs (Simpson's rule) [15 - 19]. LVEF $\geq$ 55% is generally considered as normal. However, the most recent recommendation of the American Society of echocardiography and the European Association of Cardiovascular Imaging, LVEF <52% in men and <54% in women should be considered as abnormal LVEF [14].

Visual Estimation of LVEF

For the longest time, estimation of LVEF was dependent on the eyeballing of experienced and well-trained cardiologists [20]. Several studies tested the accuracy of the visual estimation of LV and demonstrated good correlation with nuclear medicine and echo quantification [21, 22]. However, eyeball estimation requires experience and is limited by arrhythmia and extremes of heart rate and left ventricular size in addition to subjectivity. The use of visual estimation for assessment of LVEF is not recommended [14]. Therefore, several quantitative techniques have been developed to overcome these limitations.

Quantification Methods of LVEF Assessment

Tiechholz formula is one of the earliest methods for quantification of LVEF. It is based on the cube formula to calculate LV volume, which is obtained from a linear measurement form single plane. It is based on the assumption that the LV is a sphere and hence the formula uses a correction factor to correct for non-spherical qualities of the LV. According to this formula, LV Volume = $[7/(2.4 + LVID)] * LVID^3$, subsequently LVEF can be calculated form LV systolic and diastolic volumes [23]. Teichholz method provides a rapid an accurate method of LVEF quantification as it correlates well to angiographic assessment [13, 24]. Similarly, Dumesnil's method of LVEF assessment utilizes the Teichholz formula for calculating of LV diastolic volume but calculates the LV stroke volume form Doppler flow of the left ventricular outflow tract [25]. According to this formula, $SV = \pi*(LVOT/2)^2*VTI$ and therefore LVEF= (SV/ LV end-diastolic volume)*100. Quinones equation calculates LVEF by averaging multiple LV end-systolic and end-diastolic dimensions and adding a correcting factor for apical contractility [26]. A simplified version of the equation was proposed. In this equation LVEF= $(LVEDD^2-LVESD^2)/LVEDD^2*100+K$.

The K is the correction factor for apical contractility: normal=+10%, hypokinetic= 5%, akinetic=0%, dyskinetic=-5% and aneurismal=-10%. All of these methods are based on a linear measuring from a single plane and therefore their use may lead to inaccurate assessment of ejection fraction particularly patients with regional wall motion abnormalities.

Nowadays, the recommended method of LVEF quantification is the biplane method of discs or modified Simpson's rule [14]. According to this rule, the LV volume can be measured by calculating the volume of smaller ellipsoid cylinders extending form the base to the apex of the LV. The small cylinders can adapt to the regional configuration of the LV and therefore correcting for the regional wall motion abnormalities. In addition it is free of any geometric assumption. In this method the endocardial border of the LV are traced in the two and four chamber apical views in both end-diastole and end-systole, thereafter the LV volume and LVEF are calculated. The method has been shown to be very accurate in experimental and clinical models [27 - 29]. However, its utility is limited by acoustic window, body habitus and possibility of foreshortening of the LV long axis. In addition the ability of defining the endocardial border, a crucial component of the method, maybe challenging in some cases. The use of echo contrast can significantly improve the endocardial definition and therefore improve the accuracy of LVEF calculation [30] (Fig. **2**). Contrast significantly decreased uninterpretable studies form almost 12% to less than 1% [31]. Furthermore, contrast helps in identification of LV thrombus, which is a known complication of heart failure with reduced ejection fraction [31]. Although, there is a blackbox warning from the American Food and Drug Administration (FDA) regarding the use of echo contrast agents in patients with pulmonary hypertension or unstable cardiopulmonary conditions, multiple studies have demonstrated the safety of contrast agents in these conditions [32, 33].

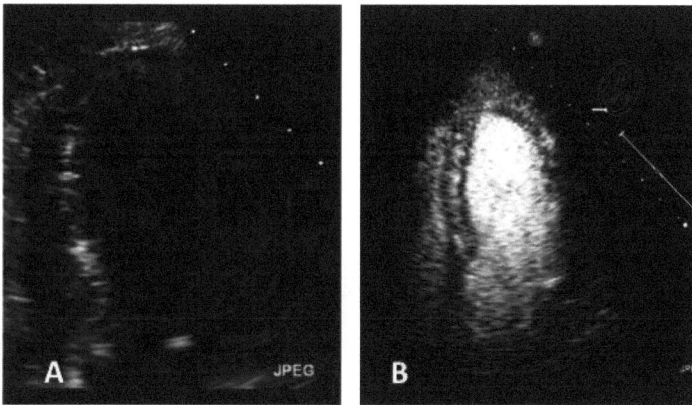

Fig. (2). Apical 4 chamber view before (A) and after (B) administration of contrast for opacification of the LV demonstrating the value of contrast in delineation of the endocardial border of the LV.

3-Dimesional echo represents a major milestone in the development of echo. It has several advantages when compared to 2D echo. 3D echo improves the visualization of the long axis of the LV eliminating the chance of foreshortening long axis of the LV and therefore the need for geometric assumption (Fig. **3**). Hence, it is proven to be an accurate and reproducible method for evaluation of LV volumes EF and mass [34 - 36]. This is particularly useful in patients with congenital heart disease as well as patients receiving chemotherapy where precise assessment of LVEF is crucial in adjustment of chemotherapeutic agents. Chemotherapy associated LV dysfunction is defined as drop in the LVEF of > 10% in asymptomatic patients and >5% in symptomatic patients [37]. In patients with undergoing chemotherapy for cancer, non-contrast 3D echo was shown to be the most reproducible technique in sequential evaluation of the LVEF and volumes over one year [36]. In addition, 3D echo provides a comprehensive assessment of regional wall motion and dyssynchrony [38]. Thus, it can help in predicting as well as following up the response to cardiac resynchronization therapy [39, 40]. Finally, 3D echo provides a real view of the valves and better quantification of valvular lesions. This is notably important in the evaluation of mitral valve, which has a complex 3D saddle shape [41, 42]. However, despite the promises of 3D echo, its use is limited by reduced temporal and spatial resolution [43].

Despite the accuracy and reproducibility of these methods, the LVEF assessment is limited by inadequate measurement and tracing of the LV and significant inter-observer variability in addition to the inherent limitation of LVEF being volume and load dependent [44]. Furthermore, it is important to understand that although LVEF is used to identify the patients with heart failure, it is considered to be a suboptimal measure of LV systolic function since it does not correlate to symptoms, functional capacity or maximal oxygen consumption [45 - 47]. Similarly, LVEF alone is not an indication for cardiac transplant [46]. Additionally, LVEF is maintained in patients with significant mitral regurgitation despite reduced stroke volume. Therefore, LVEF should be taken in consideration only within the context of the clinical presentation of the patient.

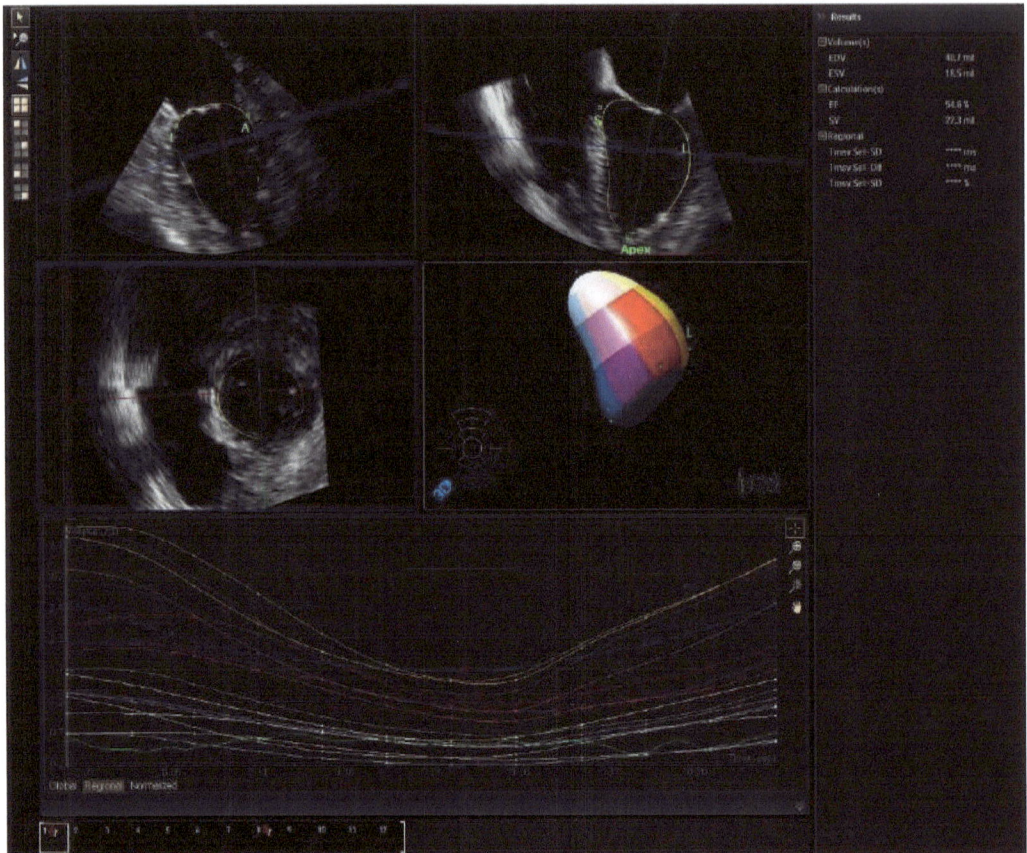

Fig. (3). 3D echo showing images. The LV endocardial borders are traced at end-diastole and end-systole to produce 3D volume and segmentation. The synchrony is of LV segments is also evaluated (lower box).

Myocardial Performance Index

Myocardial performance index (Tei index) is a measure of LV systolic function that incorporates both systolic and diastolic function and works independently of load status and geometric assumptions. It is simple, reproducible and since it is measured from Doppler signal it can be obtained even in poor image quality [48].

Tei index was validated and demonstrated significant correlation with invasive measurement of LV function (dp/dt) [49]. It has been proposed as a measure of LV function in a variety of cardiac diseases including cardiomyopathy, congenital heart disease, valvular heart disease and follow up of patients post cardiac transplant.

Tie index was first proposed by Tei *et al* in 1995 [50]. The index is presented as an absolute number and derived from calculation based on Doppler interrogation during echo study. Employing the concept LV dysfunction results in prolongation off both isovolumic times, the Tei index = (Isovolumic contraction time + Isovolumic relaxation times)/ LV ejection time. Since the isovolumic times equal the mitral valve opening time – LV ejection time, this equation can be simplified so that Tei index = (Mitral valve opening- LV ejection time)/ LV ejection time (Fig. **4**). The mean normal value of the Tei index is 0.39 ± 0.05 and it is inversely related to LVEF [50].

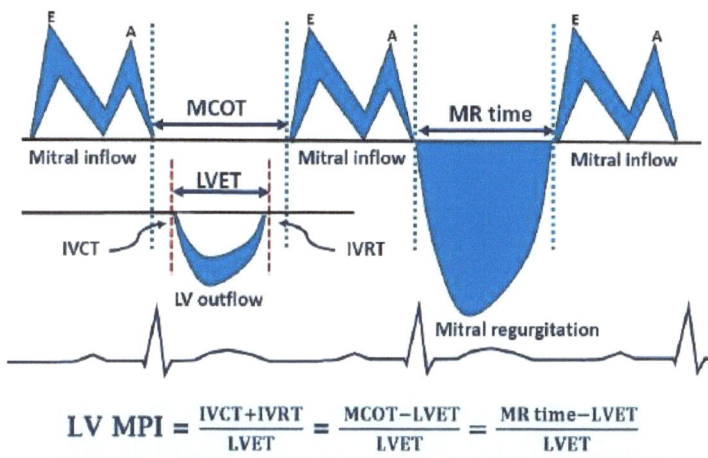

$$LV\ MPI = \frac{IVCT+IVRT}{LVET} = \frac{MCOT-LVET}{LVET} = \frac{MR\ time-LVET}{LVET}$$

Fig. (4). Calculation of LV Myocardial Performance Index (*Tei Index*) from Doppler interrogation of the mitral inflow and LV outflow tract. In the presence of mitral regurgitation, the regurgitation signal is used to calculate mitral valve opening to closure time.

Since the Tei index depends the isovolumic times, it may be considered as a surrogate of LV contractile function by reflecting repolarization and depolarization of the myocardial cells. Isovolumic contraction and relaxation times correspond to Calcium influx and exit from the myocardial cells. Therefore, Tei index is superior to LVEF in detecting early stages of LV dysfunction [51]. Similarly, it has better sensitivity in detecting LV dysfunction early after myocardial infarction [52]. Moreover, it has been shown to be of value in predicting response to therapy in patients with heart failure [53].

Nonetheless, the Tei index has its own limitations. In patients with severe diastolic dysfunction and normal systolic function, the Tei index can be normal while this group is known to have poor outcome [54]. In addition, there is technical difficulty in obtaining accurate measurement in patients with atrial arrhythmia. Finally, the use of Tei index has not been tested in large studies.

NONINVASIVE MEASUREMENT OF HEMODYNAMIC

The Doppler interrogation during echo study can provide quantitative means of measuring cardiac hemodynamic noninvasively. Several hemodynamic parameters of both the left and right ventricle can be reliably obtained from routine echo studies even in the presence of decompensated heart failure [55].

Employing the principles of fluid dynamics and echo ability to measure cardiac orifices, left ventricular stroke volume can be measured from the Doppler interrogation of the left ventricular outflow tract (LVOT). The LVOT area = ? $(D/2)^2$ and therefore the LV stroke volume can be calculated by multiplying the velocity time integral of the LVOT and LVOT area (SV= VTI_{LVOT} *? $(D/2)^2$). Subsequently, cardiac output can be calculated by multiplying the stroke volume by the heart rate (Cardiac output= SV * heart rate) [56] (Fig. **5**). Left atrial (LA) and filling pressure can also be estimated form the Doppler study. In patient with normal ejection fraction LA pressure is considered to be high if E/e′ ≥ 13, while LA pressure is normal when E/e′ ≤ 8 (where E is the early mitral inflow velocity and e′ is early mitral annular velocity) [56].

The right atrial pressure (RAP) on the other hand can be estimated from studying the inferior vena cava (IVC). The estimation is based on the size and inspiratory collapsibility of the IVC. Normal diameter (≤ 2.1 cm) and inspiratory collapse (>50%) indicates RAP of 3 mmHg (range, 0-5 mmHg), Dilated IVC (≥ 2.1 cm) with reduced respiratory variation (<50%) corresponds to RAP of 15 mmHg (range, 10-20 mmHg) and IVC diameter and respiratory variation unfitting the previous paradigm indicates RAP of 8 mmHg (range, 5-10 mmHg) [57]. Since substantial numbers of normal subjects have mild degree of tricuspid and pulmonic valve regurgitation, right ventricular (RV) pressure as well as pulmonary artery pressure could be estimated. The RV pressure can be estimated from the jet of the tricuspid regurgitation according to modified Bernoulli equation $(P=4*V^2)$, subsequently, in the absence of pulmonic valve stenosis, the systolic pulmonary pressure is calculated by adding the estimated RA pressure to the RV pressure [57]. Similarly, the diastolic pulmonary artery pressure can be estimated from the pressure of the end of the regurgitation jet of the pulmonic valve after adding the estimated the RA pressure [58] (Fig. **6**).

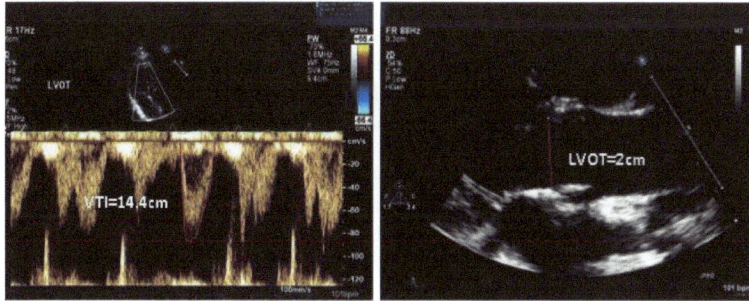

Calculation of Cardiac output

Stroke Volume (SV) = LVOT area * VTI_{LVOT}

$= \pi (D/2)^2 * VTI_{LVOT}$

$= 3.14*(2/2)^2*14.4$

$= 45$ mL

Cardiac Output = SV * Heart rate

$= 45 * 100$

$= 4500$ mL (4.5 L)

Fig. (5). Calculation of Cardiac Output by LVOT area and Doppler interrogation of LVOT.

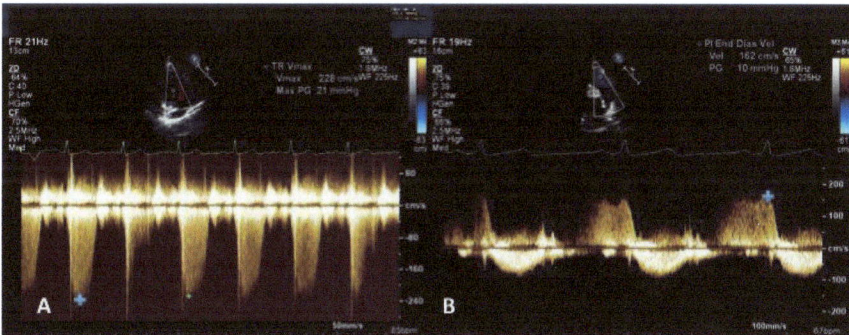

Estimation of Pulmonary Artery Pressure from Doppler study of Tricuspid Regurgitation

Systolic PA pressure = RVSP + RA Pressure (Based on IVC size and collapsibility)

$= 21 + 8$

$= 29$ mmHg

Estimation of Pulmonary Artery Pressure from Doppler study of Pulmonary regurgitation

Diastolic PA pressure = PA end-diastolic pressure + RA pressure

$= 10 + 8$

$= 18$ mmHg

Fig. (6). Estimation of Systolic and Diastolic pulmonary Artery Pressure from Doppler study of tricuspid and pulmonary valve regurgitation.

CARDIAC MECHANICS AND LV SYSTOLIC FUNCTION

In recent years, strain and strain rate have emerged as reliable and reproducible tools for assessment of LV function and contractility [59]. In addition to the advantages of tissue Doppler, independence of load, geometric assumption and to some extent operator, they are also free of the effect of tethering from the adjacent tissues. Strain and strain rates are measures of deformation, which is a better tool for detection of regional myocardial dysfunction compared to wall motion [60, 61].

Myocardial strain occurs in three direction, longitudinal, circumferential and radial (Fig. **7**) [62]. Longitudinal LV mechanics are the most vulnerable and most sensitive to the presence of myocardial disease [7]. The myocardial deformation is negative longitudinally and circumferentially and positive radially, therefore, the normal value of longitudinal strain varies between −15% and −20%, circumferential strain, −20% and −25% and radial strain 30% and 40% [63, 64]. However, the values vary among publication and highly dependent of the equipment vendor [65, 66].

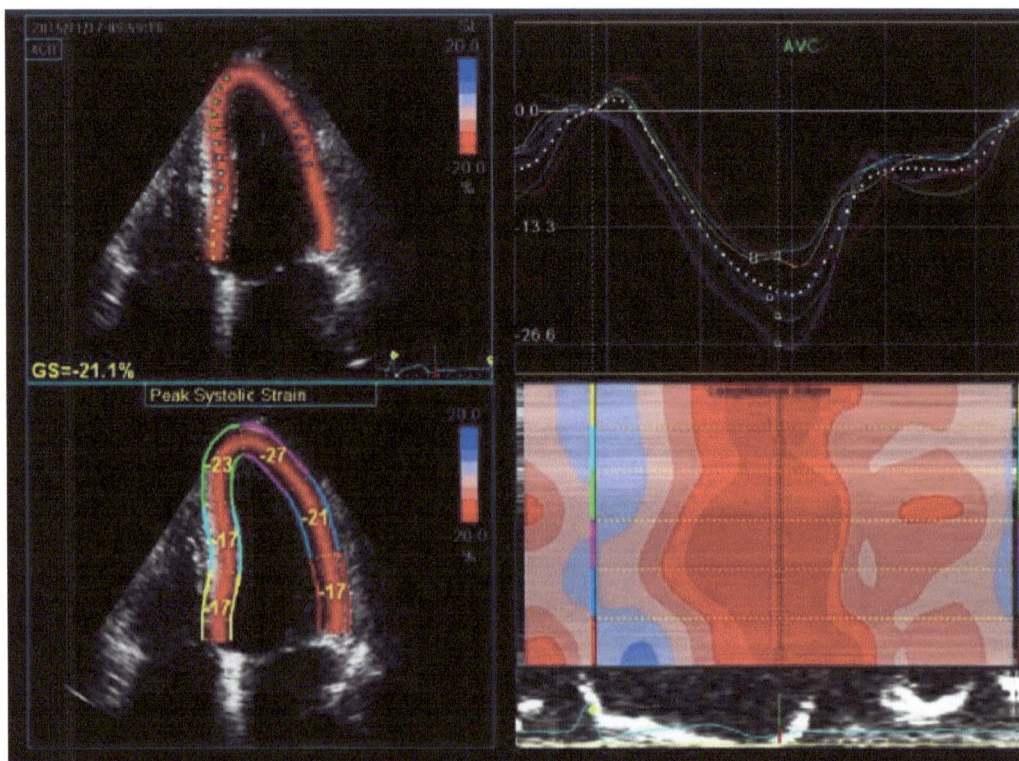

Fig. (7). Longitudinal strain or the LV as measured from the apical 4 chamber view.

The attractiveness of strain and strain rate comes from its ability to provide diagnostic and prognostic information in a variety of cardiac condition. In normal subjects, global longitudinal stain was superior to LVEF and wall motion score index in predicting all-cause mortality [67]. Similarly, global longitudinal and circumferential strain were predictive of cardiac events in patients with heart failure [68]. Global longitudinal strain was also shown to be strongly associated to a higher severity disease status in patients with heart failure [69]. Furthermore, Global longitudinal strain can detect preclinical LV dysfunction earlier than LVEF in patients receiving chemotherapy [70, 71]. Although a value of exceeding -20% is considered abnormal [71], it is important to compare the change to baseline due to significant baseline variability [71]. A change in the global longitudinal strain of > 15% is considered as the cutoff to detect cardio-toxicity [37, 71].

REGIONAL LV SYSTOLIC FUNCTION

Wall motion score index (WMSI) is a semi-quantitative of regional and global LV systolic function. In this method, the LV systolic function is determined by wall motion analysis of the LV based on the AHA17-segment heart model [72]. The distribution of these segments follows the coronary artery perfusion territory and hence the analysis can help in diagnosis of coronary artery disease [72, 73]. The wall motion is scored visually in each segment as 1 for normal contraction or hyperkinesis, 2 for hypokinesis, 3 for akinesis, 4 for dyskinesis, and 5 for aneurysmal segments [74]. The score index is derived as a sum of all scores divided by the number of segments visualized (Fig. **8**). The WMSI-derived EF has been validated against 3D echo and longitudinal strain [75 - 77]. The index was also shown to predict cardiac mortality in a large cohort of patients [78].

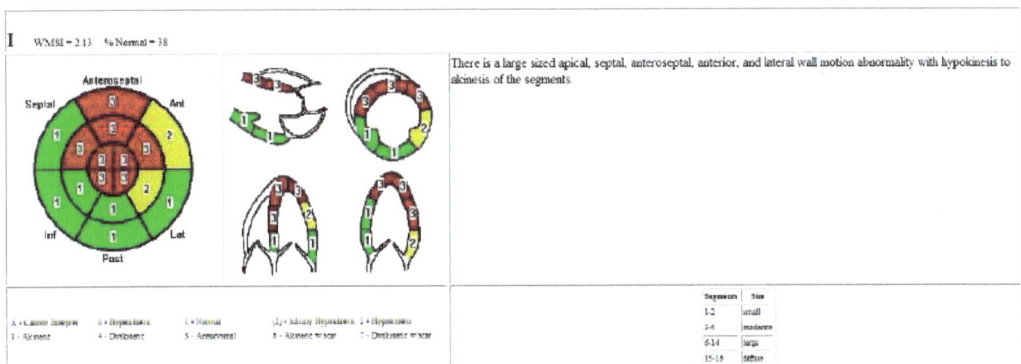

Fig. (8). Wall Motion Score Index in a patient with old anterior myocardial infarction.

ECHOCARDIOGRAPHY AND DIASTOLIC DYSFUNCTION

Heart failure with preserved ejection fraction accounts for almost half cases of heart failure [79, 80], moreover, all patients with systolic dysfunction have some degree of diastolic dysfunction. Echo remains the fundamental part of diagnosis, evaluation and grading of diastolic dysfunction [81]. In addition, patients with isolated diastolic dysfunction can progress to develop systolic heart failure [82]. According to Doppler data from the mitral and pulmonic valves, tissue Doppler and LA, diastolic dysfunction is classified into 3 grades; impaired LV relaxation, pseudo-normalization and restrictive physiology [6]. The determination of the grade of diastolic function is based on the study of the pulse Doppler of the mitral valve inflow, early filling (E wave) and atrial contraction (A wave), TDI of the septal and lateral annulus of the mitral valve (septal and lateral e′ with supplementary information from the pulmonic valve Doppler interrogation and left atrial volume.

Impaired LV relaxation, mild diastolic dysfunction, is characterized by mitral E/A ratio of < 8, E/e′ ≤ 8 and deceleration time of > 200 mS, while pseudo-normalization, moderate diastolic dysfunction, is characterized by E/A of 0.8 -1.5, E/e′ of 9-12 and deceleration time of 160-200 mS. The severe grade of diastolic dysfunction, restrictive physiology, has E/A of ≥2, E/e′ of ≥13 and deceleration time of <160 mS [6]. Estimation of LA and filling pressures were discusses earlier in this chapter. It has been shown that LA pressure estimation by E/e′ performs better than BNP in detecting volume overload [83, 84]. In addition, the severity of diastolic dysfunction provides further prognostication in patients with heart failure. The presence of restrictive physiology despite optimal medical therapy in patients with systolic heart failure, indicates poor prognosis [85]. Unfortunately, tachycardia, significant mitral pathology and ventricular pacing limit evaluation of diastolic dysfunction according in this paradigm [44].

Although the diagnosis of heart failure with preserved ejection fraction is based on the finding of normal ejection fraction in patients with heart failure, it is important to keep in mind that the LV systolic function is not entirely normal in these patients, Newer technologies such as strain and strain rate may shed further light on the degree of systolic dysfunction in this group of patients with heart failure.

LV VOLUME SHAPE AND MASS

Cardiac remodeling is a progressive process in patients with heart failure irrespective of etiology. It can be in the form of regional or global dilatation, change in the shape or alteration in the LV mass [86]. Remodeling of the LV has been shown to be of prognostic importance in many cardiac diseases. Echo provides sufficient data on the presence and extent of the remodeling in most of the cases.

Remodeling process after myocardial infarction usually results in either global dilatation or region change in the shape of the heart [87]. The extent of LV remodeling after myocardial infarction is determined by multiple factors [88, 89]. LV dilatation by echo has been shown to be associated with poor outcome post myocardial infarction [79, 90]. Similarly, change of the heart shape to become spherical is associated with poor outcome [91, 92].

The LV responds to pressure overload by increasing the thickness of the wall and therefore increasing the LV mass, which results in concentric LV hypertrophy. Volume overload on the other hand, leads to LV dilatation with resultant increase in LV mass, eccentric LV hypertrophy [93]. In patients with heart failure, LV mass is associated with increased mortality independent of LVEF [94]. Echo is an accurate and reproducible tool for assessment of LV mass [4]. However, since the mass is calculated form linear measurement from echo, it is subjective to the same limitation of measuring LV volume.

Left atrial (LA) dilatation is the end process of increased filling pressure. It provides a marker for the chronicity of heart failure process and high the chronicity of filling pressure. LA volume is considered an important prognostic value in patients with heart failure [95, 96]. LA volume can be reliably calculated from echo by biplane area length equation; LA dilatation ≥ 34 ml/m^2 is considered as the cutoff for the LA dilatation [4].

STRESS ECHOCARDIOGRAPHY

Coronary artery disease remains the most common cause of LV systolic heart failure [97]. In heart failure due to ischemic heart disease, the abnormality of myocardial contractility could represent stunning, hibernation or infarction or combination of these abnormalities [98]. Differentiation between these processes is a crucial step in decision of revascularization. Stress echocardiography is a reliable method for evaluation of myocardial viability.

Pharmacological stress echo with Dobutmine is used to detect myocardial ischemia and assess for myocardial viability [99]. During the test, images are obtained at rest and at peak Dobutamine infusion (maximum stress). Three patterns could be seen during stress echo; normal, ischemic and viable myocardium. In normal response, a normal segment either remains normal or become hyperkinetic. In the ischemic response, segmental wall motion worsens with increasing dose of Dubtamine bur get better with low dose, a phenomenon called biphasic response [100]. Akinetic segments that improve with Dobutamine are considered viable. The presence of contractile reserve in a segment indicates the viability of at least 50% of myocardial cells in that segment [101].

The prognostic value of stress echo in predicting improvement of LVEF after coronary artery bypass surgery was similar to that of PET [102]. In one study, sensitivity and specificity of dobutamine echocardiography for predicting recovery of regional function after revascularization was 84% and 81% respectively [103]. It has also been shown that the presence of contractile reserves is associated better outcome in patients with dilated cardiomyopathy [104, 105]. Furthermore, stress echo shows promising results in patients with normal LVEF and inconclusive diastolic parameters [106]. However, the accuracy of stress echo in predicting viability is limited by resting tachycardia, severe reduction of blood flow due to severe coronary artery disease and tethering effect from adjacent normal segments.

ECHOCARDIOGRAPHY AND ASSESSMENT OF THE RIGHT VENTRICLE

Multiple studies have demonstrated the prognostic value of right ventricular (RV) function in patients with heart failure [107 - 109]. The complex and 3-dimentional morphology of the RV within the chest limit the role of echo in the assessment of RV systolic function. Nonetheless, multiple echo parameters have been proven to be reliable in assessing RV function. The most commonly used parameters in assessment of RV function are tricuspid annular plane systolic excursion (TAPSE), 2D Fractional area change (FAC), RV myocardial performance index (RIMP) and tissue Doppler–derived tricuspid lateral annular systolic velocity (S′) [57].

Since it is measured from lateral tricuspid annulus, TAPSE is a measure of RV longitudinal function, but correlates well to global RV function. TAPSE < 16 mm indicates RV systolic dysfunction. 2D FAC% is obtained by planimetry of the RV in diastole and systole. Subsequently, RV systolic function is calculated as $[(FAC_{diastole}-FACsystole)/FAC_{diastole}]*100$, FAC < 35% indicates RV systolic dysfunction. TDI derived S′ velocity < 10 cm/s also indicates RV systolic dysfunction. Finally, RIMP is measured similar to Tei index for the LV, RIMP > 0.40 by pulsed Doppler and > 0.55 by tissue Doppler is considered abnormal [57, 110 - 112]. Strain and strain rate have been studied in assessment of RV function, however lack of normal value and the small sample size in the studies examining their performance limit it's their use in daily clinical practice.

These parameters have been proven to be of prognostic value in various cardiac conditions. FAC% is shown to be an independent predictor of heart failure and sudden cardiac death post pulmonary embolism and myocardial infarction [113 -

115]. RIMP has been shown to have prognostic value in pulmonary hypertension, hypertrophic cardiomyopathy and congenital heart disease [116 - 119]. Finally RV strain and strain rate were also shown to have incremental prognostic value in predicting death and cardiac transplant in patients with chronic heart failure [120].

ECHOCARDIOGRAPHY AND ETIOLOGY OF HEART FAILURE

Echocardiography is usually the imaging step in the evaluation of patients with heart failure. Initial findings can help differentiate between different etiologies of heart failure. Regional wall motion abnormalities suggest ischemic heart disease, albeit sometimes can be seen in cardiomyopathy. LV hypertrophy suggests hypertension as a cause of heart failure, while asymmetrical hypertrophy indicates hypertrophic cardiomyopathy. Certain cardiac conditions, like amyloidosis has pathognomonic appearance on echo. Valvular heart diseases are among the commonest etiology of heart failure [121]. Echo is a fundamental investigation in the evaluation and management of valvular heart disease [5, 122]. Evaluation of mitral valve regurgitation is particularly important since it can be a cause or a consequence of functional mitral regurgitation of heart failure [123, 124]. Constrictive pericarditis presents with symptoms similar to those of heart failure. Echo can reliably diagnose and provide hemodynamic assessment of constrictive pericarditis [125, 126].

ECHOCARDIOGRAPHY IN MANAGEMENT AND PROGNOSIS OF HEART FAILURE

In addition to its role in the diagnosis of heart failure, echo provides important information to guide pharmacological and device therapy as well as prognosis. Initiation and escalation of medication in heart failure are dependent on patient symptoms and LVEF assessed by echocardiography. Angiotensin converting enzyme inhibitor (ACEi), Angiontensin receptor blockers (ARB), beta-blockers and aldosterone antagonists are the main stay of treatment of patients with heart failure and reduced ejection fraction. These medications are known to reverse adverse cardiac remodeling and improve survival [1]. Echo is routinely used as a follow up tool for the assessment of LVEF after initiation of these medications and is used to measure response to medication [127]. In patients on cardio-toxic chemotherapy for cancer, echo is used to assess changes in LVEF and therefore prevent further deterioration of LVEF either by stopping the cardio-toxic medication or decreasing the dose [128].

Echocardiography and Selection of Patients for Device Therapy

Cardiac arrhythmia particularly ventricular fibrillation (VF) is a common cause of mortality in patients with heart failure and reduced ejection fraction [129, 130].

Implantable Cardioverter-defibrillator (AICD) implantation for primary prevention has been shown to very efficacious in prevention of sudden cardiac death in patients with low EF. Multiple studies have shown the benefit of AICD for primary prevention in patients with LVEF≤35% despite medical therapy regardless of etiology of heart failure [131 - 133]. Echo remains the first step in evaluation of patients prior to AICD implantation.

Cardiac dyssynchrony is prevalent in many patients with heart failure. The loss of coordination between LV myocardial segments results in impairment of cardiac output and therefore worsening of heart failure symptoms [134]. Cardiac resynchronization therapy (CRT) was proven to improve heart failure symptoms and survival [135]. It was also shown to reverse the adverse remodeling processes in heart failure. CRT was also proven to be associated with significant reduction in LV volumes and severity of mitral regurgitation [136 - 138]. CRT is indicated in patients with symptomatic heart failure, LVEF ≤ 35% and wide QRS complexes on electrocardiogram [139]. In addition to assessment of LVEF, echo can provide useful information on the degree location and extent of dyssynchrony. Dyssynchrony can be evaluated by tissue Doppler or more recently by strain and strain rate [140, 141]. In addition to patient selection, echo is used to assess response to CRT after implantation [139, 142].

Mechanical circulatory support in heart failure is rapidly evolving. In recent years, the use of ventricular assessed device in patients with heart failure is increasing either as a bridge to transplant or destination therapy [143]. Echo is fundamental in patient selection as well as follow-up of these devices [144]. Echo can provide information on whether the patient requires left ventricular or bi-ventricular assessed device [145]. Echo also detects the presence of intra-cardiac shunt [146], which needs to be corrected before implantation. Furthermore, echo is also used to detect complication of these devices such as thrombus, LVOT obstruction or valvular of insufficiency [147, 148].

Echocardiography and Early Detection of Heart Failure

American College of Cardiology and American Heart Association have proposed four stages of heart failure based on the presence of risk factor and heart failure symptoms [149]. According to this staging system, stage A and B represent early stages of heart failure before development of symptoms. Screening of patients in these stages is an important step in early detection and therefore prevention of heart failure. With the aging world population and increased incidence of hypertension and diabetes, which are risk factors for development of heart failure [150], echo represents a cost-effective and reliable in initial evaluation and follows up of these patients.

CONCLUSION

Although no single imaging modality provides all the needed information in heart failure, echocardiography remains imperative in heart failure management. Echo is considered the first and most widely available modality in the evaluation of heart failure. Furthermore, it has a superior role in the evaluation of heart failure due to valvular heart disease and it provides adequate and reliable information on diagnosis, therapeutic options and prognosis in all the stages of heart failure. 3D-echo has a superior role in the evaluation of the LV and RV volume and provides better assessment of regional wall motion abnormalities. In addition, it has a pivotal role in the assessment of mitral and aortic valve pathology. Cardiac mechanics with speckle tracking has great potentials in assessment of subclinical LV systolic dysfunction particularly in patients receiving chemotherapy. It also has potential in the assessment of certain cardiomyopathy such as amyliodosis. Albeit more than 60 years old, echo has promising new application with uncharted frontiers particularly in the field of 3D imaging and cardiac mechanics.

CONSENT FOR PUBLICATION

Not applicable.

CONFLICT OF INTEREST

The authors confirm that this chapter contents have no conflict of interest.

ACKNOWLEDGEMENTS

Declared none.

REFERENCES

[1]	Yancy CW, Jessup M, Bozkurt B, *et al.* 2013 ACCF/AHA guideline for the management of heart failure: a report of the American College of Cardiology Foundation/American Heart Association Task Force on practice guidelines. Circulation 2013; 128(16): e240-327.
[http://dx.doi.org/10.1161/CIR.0b013e31829e8776] [PMID: 23741058]

[2]	McMurray JJ, Adamopoulos S, Anker SD, *et al.* ESC Guidelines for the diagnosis and treatment of acute and chronic heart failure 2012: The Task Force for the Diagnosis and Treatment of Acute and Chronic Heart Failure 2012 of the European Society of Cardiology. Developed in collaboration with the Heart Failure Association (HFA) of the ESC. Eur Heart J 2012; 33(14): 1787-847.
[http://dx.doi.org/10.1093/eurheartj/ehs104] [PMID: 22611136]

[3]	Baumgartner H, Hung J, Bermejo J, *et al.* Echocardiographic assessment of valve stenosis: EAE/ASE recommendations for clinical practice. J Am Soc Echocardiogr 2009; 22(1): 1-23.
[http://dx.doi.org/10.1016/j.echo.2008.11.029] [PMID: 19130998]

[4]	Lang RM, *et al.* Recommendations for cardiac chamber quantification by echocardiography in adults: An update from the American Society of Echocardiography and the European Association of Cardiovascular Imaging J Am Soc Echocardiogr 2015; 28(1): 1-39. e14

[5]   Zoghbi WA, Enriquez-Sarano M, Foster E, *et al.* Recommendations for evaluation of the severity of native valvular regurgitation with two-dimensional and Doppler echocardiography. J Am Soc Echocardiogr 2003; 16(7): 777-802.
[http://dx.doi.org/10.1016/S0894-7317(03)00335-3] [PMID: 12835667]

[6]   Nagueh SF, Appleton CP, Gillebert TC, *et al.* Recommendations for the evaluation of left ventricular diastolic function by echocardiography. J Am Soc Echocardiogr 2009; 22(2): 107-33.
[http://dx.doi.org/10.1016/j.echo.2008.11.023] [PMID: 19187853]

[7]   Mor-Avi V, Lang RM, Badano LP, *et al.* Current and evolving echocardiographic techniques for the quantitative evaluation of cardiac mechanics: ASE/EAE consensus statement on methodology and indications endorsed by the Japanese Society of Echocardiography. J Am Soc Echocardiogr 2011; 24(3): 277-313.
[http://dx.doi.org/10.1016/j.echo.2011.01.015] [PMID: 21338865]

[8]   Otto CM. The practice of clinical echocardiography. Philadelphia, PA: Elsevier/Saunders 2012.

[9]   Maciver DH. The relative impact of circumferential and longitudinal shortening on left ventricular ejection fraction and stroke volume. Exp Clin Cardiol 2012; 17(1): 5-11.
[PMID: 23204893]

[10]   Richardson P, McKenna W, Bristow M, *et al.* Report of the 1995 World Health Organization/ International Society and Federation of Cardiology Task Force on the Definition and Classification of cardiomyopathies. Circulation 1996; 93(5): 841-2.
[http://dx.doi.org/10.1161/01.CIR.93.5.841] [PMID: 8598070]

[11]   Lang RM, Bierig M, Devereux RB, *et al.* Chamber Quantification Writing Group; American Society of Echocardiography's Guidelines and Standards Committee; European Association of Echocardiography. Recommendations for chamber quantification: a report from the American Society of Echocardiography's Guidelines and Standards Committee and the Chamber Quantification Writing Group, developed in conjunction with the European Association of Echocardiography, a branch of the European Society of Cardiology. J Am Soc Echocardiogr 2005; 18(12): 1440-63.
[http://dx.doi.org/10.1016/j.echo.2005.10.005] [PMID: 16376782]

[12]   Lang RM, Borow KM, Neumann A, Janzen D. Systemic vascular resistance: an unreliable index of left ventricular afterload. Circulation 1986; 74(5): 1114-23.
[http://dx.doi.org/10.1161/01.CIR.74.5.1114] [PMID: 3769169]

[13]   Weyman AE. Principles and practice of echocardiography. 2nd ed., Philadelphia: Lea & Febiger. xvii 1994.

[14]   Lang RM, Badano LP, Mor-Avi V, *et al.* Recommendations for cardiac chamber quantification by echocardiography in adults: an update from the American Society of Echocardiography and the European Association of Cardiovascular Imaging. Eur Heart J Cardiovasc Imaging 2015; 16(3): 233-70.
[http://dx.doi.org/10.1093/ehjci/jev014] [PMID: 25712077]

[15]   Hermann HJ, Bartle SH. Left ventricular volumes by angiocardiography: comparison of methods and simplification of techniques. Cardiovasc Res 1968; 2(4): 404-14.
[http://dx.doi.org/10.1093/cvr/2.4.404] [PMID: 5727771]

[16]   Sandler H, Dodge HT. The use of single plane angiocardiograms for the calculation of left ventricular volume in man. Am Heart J 1968; 75(3): 325-34.
[http://dx.doi.org/10.1016/0002-8703(68)90089-6] [PMID: 5638471]

[17]   Davila JC, Sanmarco ME. An analysis of the fit of mathematical models applicable to the measurement of left ventricular volume. Am J Cardiol 1966; 18(1): 31-42.
[http://dx.doi.org/10.1016/0002-9149(66)90193-7] [PMID: 5938909]

[18]   Chapman CB, Baker O, Reynolds J, Bonte FJ. Use of biplane cinefluorography for measurement of ventricular volume. Circulation 1958; 18(6): 1105-17.

[http://dx.doi.org/10.1161/01.CIR.18.6.1105] [PMID: 13608839]

[19] Belenkie I, Nutter DO, Clark DW, McCraw DB, Raizner AE. Assessment of left ventricular dimensions and function by echocardiography. Am J Cardiol 1973; 31(6): 755-62.
[http://dx.doi.org/10.1016/0002-9149(73)90011-8] [PMID: 4706732]

[20] Foster E, Cahalan MK. The search for intelligent quantitation in echocardiography: "eyeball," "trackball" and beyond. J Am Coll Cardiol 1993; 22(3): 848-50.
[http://dx.doi.org/10.1016/0735-1097(93)90201-B] [PMID: 8354822]

[21] Stamm RB, Carabello BA, Mayers DL, Martin RP. Two-dimensional echocardiographic measurement of left ventricular ejection fraction: prospective analysis of what constitutes an adequate determination. Am Heart J 1982; 104(1): 136-44.
[http://dx.doi.org/10.1016/0002-8703(82)90651-2] [PMID: 7090969]

[22] Amico AF, Lichtenberg GS, Reisner SA, Stone CK, Schwartz RG, Meltzer RS. Superiority of visual *versus* computerized echocardiographic estimation of radionuclide left ventricular ejection fraction. Am Heart J 1989; 118(6): 1259-65.
[http://dx.doi.org/10.1016/0002-8703(89)90018-5] [PMID: 2686380]

[23] Teichholz LE, Kreulen T, Herman MV, Gorlin R. Problems in echocardiographic volume determinations: echocardiographic-angiographic correlations in the presence of absence of asynergy. Am J Cardiol 1976; 37(1): 7-11.
[http://dx.doi.org/10.1016/0002-9149(76)90491-4] [PMID: 1244736]

[24] Kronik G, Slany J, Mösslacher H. Comparative value of eight M-mode echocardiographic formulas for determining left ventricular stroke volume. A correlative study with thermodilution and left ventricular single-plane cineangiography. Circulation 1979; 60(6): 1308-16.
[http://dx.doi.org/10.1161/01.CIR.60.6.1308] [PMID: 498456]

[25] Dumesnil JG, Dion D, Yvorchuk K, Davies RA, Chan K. A new, simple and accurate method for determining ejection fraction by Doppler echocardiography. Can J Cardiol 1995; 11(11): 1007-14.
[PMID: 8542542]

[26] Quinones MA, Waggoner AD, Reduto LA, *et al.* A new, simplified and accurate method for determining ejection fraction with two-dimensional echocardiography. Circulation 1981; 64(4): 744-53.
[http://dx.doi.org/10.1161/01.CIR.64.4.744] [PMID: 7273375]

[27] Erbel R, Krebs W, Henn G, *et al.* Comparison of single-plane and biplane volume determination by two-dimensional echocardiography. 1. Asymmetric model hearts. Eur Heart J 1982; 3(5): 469-80.
[http://dx.doi.org/10.1093/oxfordjournals.eurheartj.a061334] [PMID: 7173231]

[28] Mercier JC, DiSessa TG, Jarmakani JM, *et al.* Two-dimensional echocardiographic assessment of left ventricular volumes and ejection fraction in children. Circulation 1982; 65(5): 962-9.
[http://dx.doi.org/10.1161/01.CIR.65.5.962] [PMID: 7074761]

[29] Wahr DW, Wang YS, Schiller NB. Left ventricular volumes determined by two-dimensional echocardiography in a normal adult population. J Am Coll Cardiol 1983; 1(3): 863-8.
[http://dx.doi.org/10.1016/S0735-1097(83)80200-9] [PMID: 6687472]

[30] Porter TR, Abdelmoneim S, Belcik JT, *et al.* Guidelines for the cardiac sonographer in the performance of contrast echocardiography: a focused update from the American Society of Echocardiography. J Am Soc Echocardiogr 2014; 27(8): 797-810.
[http://dx.doi.org/10.1016/j.echo.2014.05.011] [PMID: 25085408]

[31] Kurt M, Shaikh KA, Peterson L, *et al.* Impact of contrast echocardiography on evaluation of ventricular function and clinical management in a large prospective cohort. J Am Coll Cardiol 2009; 53(9): 802-10.
[http://dx.doi.org/10.1016/j.jacc.2009.01.005] [PMID: 19245974]

[32] Khawaja OA, Shaikh KA, Al-Mallah MH. Meta-analysis of adverse cardiovascular events associated

with echocardiographic contrast agents. Am J Cardiol 2010; 106(5): 742-7.
[http://dx.doi.org/10.1016/j.amjcard.2010.04.034] [PMID: 20723656]

[33] Main ML, Ryan AC, Davis TE, Albano MP, Kusnetzky LL, Hibberd M. Acute mortality in hospitalized patients undergoing echocardiography with and without an ultrasound contrast agent (multicenter registry results in 4,300,966 consecutive patients). Am J Cardiol 2008; 102(12): 1742-6.
[http://dx.doi.org/10.1016/j.amjcard.2008.08.019] [PMID: 19064035]

[34] Hung J, Lang R, Flachskampf F, *et al.* 3D echocardiography: a review of the current status and future directions. J Am Soc Echocardiogr 2007; 20(3): 213-33.
[http://dx.doi.org/10.1016/j.echo.2007.01.010] [PMID: 17336747]

[35] Lang RM, Badano LP, Tsang W, *et al.* EAE/ASE recommendations for image acquisition and display using three-dimensional echocardiography. J Am Soc Echocardiogr 2012; 25(1): 3-46.
[http://dx.doi.org/10.1016/j.echo.2011.11.010] [PMID: 22183020]

[36] Thavendiranathan P, Grant AD, Negishi T, Plana JC, Popović ZB, Marwick TH. Reproducibility of echocardiographic techniques for sequential assessment of left ventricular ejection fraction and volumes: application to patients undergoing cancer chemotherapy. J Am Coll Cardiol 2013; 61(1): 77-84.
[http://dx.doi.org/10.1016/j.jacc.2012.09.035] [PMID: 23199515]

[37] Plana JC, Galderisi M, Barac A, *et al.* Expert consensus for multimodality imaging evaluation of adult patients during and after cancer therapy: a report from the American Society of Echocardiography and the European Association of Cardiovascular Imaging. J Am Soc Echocardiogr 2014; 27(9): 911-39.
[http://dx.doi.org/10.1016/j.echo.2014.07.012] [PMID: 25172399]

[38] Kapetanakis S, Kearney MT, Siva A, Gall N, Cooklin M, Monaghan MJ. Real-time three-dimensional echocardiography: a novel technique to quantify global left ventricular mechanical dyssynchrony. Circulation 2005; 112(7): 992-1000.
[http://dx.doi.org/10.1161/CIRCULATIONAHA.104.474445] [PMID: 16087800]

[39] Sonne C, Sugeng L, Takeuchi M, *et al.* Real-time 3-dimensional echocardiographic assessment of left ventricular dyssynchrony: pitfalls in patients with dilated cardiomyopathy. JACC Cardiovasc Imaging 2009; 2(7): 802-12.
[http://dx.doi.org/10.1016/j.jcmg.2009.03.012] [PMID: 19608128]

[40] Marsan NA, Bleeker GB, Ypenburg C, *et al.* Real-time three-dimensional echocardiography permits quantification of left ventricular mechanical dyssynchrony and predicts acute response to cardiac resynchronization therapy. J Cardiovasc Electrophysiol 2008; 19(4): 392-9.
[http://dx.doi.org/10.1111/j.1540-8167.2007.01056.x] [PMID: 18179529]

[41] Kahlert P, Plicht B, Schenk IM, Janosi RA, Erbel R, Buck T. Direct assessment of size and shape of noncircular vena contracta area in functional *versus* organic mitral regurgitation using real-time three-dimensional echocardiography. J Am Soc Echocardiogr 2008; 21(8): 912-21.
[http://dx.doi.org/10.1016/j.echo.2008.02.003] [PMID: 18385013]

[42] Plicht B, Kahlert P, Goldwasser R, *et al.* Direct quantification of mitral regurgitant flow volume by real-time three-dimensional echocardiography using dealiasing of color Doppler flow at the vena contracta. J Am Soc Echocardiogr 2008; 21(12): 1337-46.
[http://dx.doi.org/10.1016/j.echo.2008.09.022] [PMID: 19041578]

[43] Lang RM, Mor-Avi V, Dent JM, Kramer CM. Three-dimensional echocardiography: is it ready for everyday clinical use? JACC Cardiovasc Imaging 2009; 2(1): 114-7.
[http://dx.doi.org/10.1016/j.jcmg.2008.10.006] [PMID: 19356542]

[44] Marwick TH. The role of echocardiography in heart failure. J Nucl Med 2015; 56 (Suppl. 4): 31S-8S.
[http://dx.doi.org/10.2967/jnumed.114.150433] [PMID: 26033901]

[45] Baker BJ, Wilen MM, Boyd CM, Dinh H, Franciosa JA. Relation of right ventricular ejection fraction to exercise capacity in chronic left ventricular failure. Am J Cardiol 1984; 54(6): 596-9.
[http://dx.doi.org/10.1016/0002-9149(84)90256-X] [PMID: 6475779]

[46] Mancini DM, Eisen H, Kussmaul W, Mull R, Edmunds LH Jr, Wilson JR. Value of peak exercise oxygen consumption for optimal timing of cardiac transplantation in ambulatory patients with heart failure. Circulation 1991; 83(3): 778-86.
[http://dx.doi.org/10.1161/01.CIR.83.3.778] [PMID: 1999029]

[47] Smart N, Haluska B, Leano R, Case C, Mottram PM, Marwick TH. Determinants of functional capacity in patients with chronic heart failure: role of filling pressure and systolic and diastolic function. Am Heart J 2005; 149(1): 152-8.
[http://dx.doi.org/10.1016/j.ahj.2004.06.017] [PMID: 15660047]

[48] Kirkpatrick JN, Vannan MA, Narula J, Lang RM. Echocardiography in heart failure: applications, utility, and new horizons. J Am Coll Cardiol 2007; 50(5): 381-96.
[http://dx.doi.org/10.1016/j.jacc.2007.03.048] [PMID: 17662389]

[49] Tei C, Nishimura RA, Seward JB, Tajik AJ. Noninvasive Doppler-derived myocardial performance index: correlation with simultaneous measurements of cardiac catheterization measurements. J Am Soc Echocardiogr 1997; 10(2): 169-78.
[http://dx.doi.org/10.1016/S0894-7317(97)70090-7] [PMID: 9083973]

[50] Tei C, Ling LH, Hodge DO, *et al.* New index of combined systolic and diastolic myocardial performance: a simple and reproducible measure of cardiac function--a study in normals and dilated cardiomyopathy. J Cardiol 1995; 26(6): 357-66.
[PMID: 8558414]

[51] Arnlöv J, Ingelsson E, Risérus U, Andrén B, Lind L. Myocardial performance index, a Doppler-derived index of global left ventricular function, predicts congestive heart failure in elderly men. Eur Heart J 2004; 25(24): 2220-5.
[http://dx.doi.org/10.1016/j.ehj.2004.10.021] [PMID: 15589639]

[52] Poulsen SH, Jensen SE, Tei C, Seward JB, Egstrup K. Value of the Doppler index of myocardial performance in the early phase of acute myocardial infarction. J Am Soc Echocardiogr 2000; 13(8): 723-30.
[http://dx.doi.org/10.1067/mje.2000.105174] [PMID: 10936815]

[53] Mikkelsen KV, Møller JE, Bie P, Ryde H, Videbaek L, Haghfelt T. Tei index and neurohormonal activation in patients with incident heart failure: serial changes and prognostic value. Eur J Heart Fail 2006; 8(6): 599-608.
[http://dx.doi.org/10.1016/j.ejheart.2005.11.015] [PMID: 16469536]

[54] Nijland F, Kamp O, Karreman AJ, van Eenige MJ, Visser CA. Prognostic implications of restrictive left ventricular filling in acute myocardial infarction: a serial Doppler echocardiographic study. J Am Coll Cardiol 1997; 30(7): 1618-24.
[http://dx.doi.org/10.1016/S0735-1097(97)00369-0] [PMID: 9385885]

[55] Nagueh SF, Bhatt R, Vivo RP, *et al.* Echocardiographic evaluation of hemodynamics in patients with decompensated systolic heart failure. Circ Cardiovasc Imaging 2011; 4(3): 220-7.
[http://dx.doi.org/10.1161/CIRCIMAGING.111.963496] [PMID: 21398512]

[56] Quiñones MA, Otto CM, Stoddard M, Waggoner A, Zoghbi WA. Recommendations for quantification of Doppler echocardiography: a report from the Doppler Quantification Task Force of the Nomenclature and Standards Committee of the American Society of Echocardiography. J Am Soc Echocardiogr 2002; 15(2): 167-84.
[http://dx.doi.org/10.1067/mje.2002.120202] [PMID: 11836492]

[57] Rudski LG, Lai WW, Afilalo J, *et al.* Guidelines for the echocardiographic assessment of the right heart in adults: a report from the American Society of Echocardiography endorsed by the European Association of Echocardiography, a registered branch of the European Society of Cardiology, and the Canadian Society of Echocardiography. J Am Soc Echocardiogr 2010; 23(7): 685-713.
[http://dx.doi.org/10.1016/j.echo.2010.05.010] [PMID: 20620859]

[58] Masuyama T, Kodama K, Kitabatake A, Sato H, Nanto S, Inoue M. Continuous-wave Doppler

echocardiographic detection of pulmonary regurgitation and its application to noninvasive estimation of pulmonary artery pressure. Circulation 1986; 74(3): 484-92.
[http://dx.doi.org/10.1161/01.CIR.74.3.484] [PMID: 2943530]

[59] D'hooge J, Heimdal A, Jamal F, *et al.* Regional strain and strain rate measurements by cardiac ultrasound: principles, implementation and limitations. Eur J Echocardiogr 2000; 1(3): 154-70.
[http://dx.doi.org/10.1053/euje.2000.0031] [PMID: 11916589]

[60] Stoylen A, Heimdal A, Bjornstad K, Torp HG, Skjaerpe T. Strain Rate Imaging by Ultrasound in the Diagnosis of Regional Dysfunction of the Left Ventricle. Echocardiography 1999; 16(4): 321-9.
[http://dx.doi.org/10.1111/j.1540-8175.1999.tb00821.x] [PMID: 11175157]

[61] Urheim S, Edvardsen T, Torp H, Angelsen B, Smiseth OA. Myocardial strain by Doppler echocardiography. Validation of a new method to quantify regional myocardial function. Circulation 2000; 102(10): 1158-64.
[http://dx.doi.org/10.1161/01.CIR.102.10.1158] [PMID: 10973846]

[62] Dandel M, Lehmkuhl H, Knosalla C, Suramelashvili N, Hetzer R. Strain and strain rate imaging by echocardiography - basic concepts and clinical applicability. Curr Cardiol Rev 2009; 5(2): 133-48.
[http://dx.doi.org/10.2174/157340309788166642] [PMID: 20436854]

[63] Abduch MC, Alencar AM, Mathias W Jr, Vieira ML. Cardiac mechanics evaluated by speckle tracking echocardiography. Arq Bras Cardiol 2014; 102(4): 403-12.
[http://dx.doi.org/10.5935/abc.20140041] [PMID: 24844877]

[64] Marwick TH, Leano RL, Brown J, *et al.* Myocardial strain measurement with 2-dimensional speckle-tracking echocardiography: definition of normal range. JACC Cardiovasc Imaging 2009; 2(1): 80-4.
[http://dx.doi.org/10.1016/j.jcmg.2007.12.007] [PMID: 19356538]

[65] Kuznetsova T, Herbots L, Richart T, *et al.* Left ventricular strain and strain rate in a general population. Eur Heart J 2008; 29(16): 2014-23.
[http://dx.doi.org/10.1093/eurheartj/ehn280] [PMID: 18583396]

[66] Dalen H, Thorstensen A, Aase SA, *et al.* Segmental and global longitudinal strain and strain rate based on echocardiography of 1266 healthy individuals: the HUNT study in Norway. Eur J Echocardiogr 2010; 11(2): 176-83.
[PMID: 19946115]

[67] Stanton T, Leano R, Marwick TH. Prediction of all-cause mortality from global longitudinal speckle strain: comparison with ejection fraction and wall motion scoring. Circ Cardiovasc Imaging 2009; 2(5): 356-64.
[http://dx.doi.org/10.1161/CIRCIMAGING.109.862334] [PMID: 19808623]

[68] Cho GY, Marwick TH, Kim HS, Kim MK, Hong KS, Oh DJ. Global 2-dimensional strain as a new prognosticator in patients with heart failure. J Am Coll Cardiol 2009; 54(7): 618-24.
[http://dx.doi.org/10.1016/j.jacc.2009.04.061] [PMID: 19660692]

[69] Rangel I, Gonçalves A, de Sousa C, *et al.* Global longitudinal strain as a potential prognostic marker in patients with chronic heart failure and systolic dysfunction. Rev Port Cardiol 2014; 33(7-8): 403-9.
[http://dx.doi.org/10.1016/j.repc.2014.01.023] [PMID: 25155003]

[70] Hare JL, Brown JK, Leano R, Jenkins C, Woodward N, Marwick TH. Use of myocardial deformation imaging to detect preclinical myocardial dysfunction before conventional measures in patients undergoing breast cancer treatment with trastuzumab. Am Heart J 2009; 158(2): 294-301.
[http://dx.doi.org/10.1016/j.ahj.2009.05.031] [PMID: 19619708]

[71] Thavendiranathan P, Poulin F, Lim KD, Plana JC, Woo A, Marwick TH. Use of myocardial strain imaging by echocardiography for the early detection of cardiotoxicity in patients during and after cancer chemotherapy: a systematic review. J Am Coll Cardiol 2014; 63 (25 Pt A): 2751-68.
[http://dx.doi.org/10.1016/j.jacc.2014.01.073] [PMID: 24703918]

[72] Cerqueira MD, Weissman NJ, Dilsizian V, *et al.* Standardized myocardial segmentation and

nomenclature for tomographic imaging of the heart. A statement for healthcare professionals from the Cardiac Imaging Committee of the Council on Clinical Cardiology of the American Heart Association. Circulation 2002; 105(4): 539-42.
[http://dx.doi.org/10.1161/hc0402.102975] [PMID: 11815441]

[73]   Herman MV, Gorlin R. Implications of left ventricular asynergy. Am J Cardiol 1969; 23(4): 538-47.
[http://dx.doi.org/10.1016/0002-9149(69)90007-1] [PMID: 5781881]

[74]   Schiller NB, Shah PM, Crawford M, *et al.* Recommendations for quantitation of the left ventricle by two-dimensional echocardiography. American Society of Echocardiography Committee on Standards, Subcommittee on Quantitation of Two-Dimensional Echocardiograms. J Am Soc Echocardiogr 1989; 2(5): 358-67.
[http://dx.doi.org/10.1016/S0894-7317(89)80014-8] [PMID: 2698218]

[75]   Palmieri V, Russo C, Buonomo A, Palmieri EA, Celentano A. Novel wall motion score-based method for estimating global left ventricular ejection fraction: validation by real-time 3D echocardiography and global longitudinal strain. Eur J Echocardiogr 2010; 11(2): 125-30.
[http://dx.doi.org/10.1093/ejechocard/jep177] [PMID: 19933521]

[76]   Lebeau R, Di Lorenzo M, Amyot R, Veilleux M, Lemieux R, Sauvé C. A new tool for estimating left ventricular ejection fraction derived from wall motion score index. Can J Cardiol 2003; 19(4): 397-404.
[PMID: 12704486]

[77]   Rifkin RD, Koito H. Comparison with radionuclide angiography of two new geometric and four nongeometric models for echocardiographic estimation of left ventricular ejection fraction using segmental wall motion scoring. Am J Cardiol 1990; 65(22): 1485-90.
[http://dx.doi.org/10.1016/0002-9149(90)91360-I] [PMID: 2353656]

[78]   Devereux RB, Roman MJ, Palmieri V, *et al.* Prognostic implications of ejection fraction from linear echocardiographic dimensions: the Strong Heart Study. Am Heart J 2003; 146(3): 527-34.
[http://dx.doi.org/10.1016/S0002-8703(03)00229-1] [PMID: 12947374]

[79]   Cleland JG, Torabi A, Khan NK. Epidemiology and management of heart failure and left ventricular systolic dysfunction in the aftermath of a myocardial infarction Heart 2005; 91 (2): ii7-13. discussion ii31, ii43-8
[http://dx.doi.org/10.1136/hrt.2005.062026]

[80]   Yancy CW, Jessup M, Bozkurt B, *et al.* 2013 ACCF/AHA guideline for the management of heart failure: a report of the American College of Cardiology Foundation/American Heart Association Task Force on Practice Guidelines. J Am Coll Cardiol 2013; 62(16): e147-239.
[http://dx.doi.org/10.1016/j.jacc.2013.05.019] [PMID: 23747642]

[81]   Kane GC, Karon BL, Mahoney DW, *et al.* Progression of left ventricular diastolic dysfunction and risk of heart failure. JAMA 2011; 306(8): 856-63.
[http://dx.doi.org/10.1001/jama.2011.1201] [PMID: 21862747]

[82]   Aurigemma GP, Gottdiener JS, Shemanski L, Gardin J, Kitzman D. Predictive value of systolic and diastolic function for incident congestive heart failure in the elderly: the cardiovascular health study. J Am Coll Cardiol 2001; 37(4): 1042-8.
[http://dx.doi.org/10.1016/S0735-1097(01)01110-X] [PMID: 11263606]

[83]   Mottram PM, Leano R, Marwick TH. Usefulness of B-type natriuretic peptide in hypertensive patients with exertional dyspnea and normal left ventricular ejection fraction and correlation with new echocardiographic indexes of systolic and diastolic function. Am J Cardiol 2003; 92(12): 1434-8.
[http://dx.doi.org/10.1016/j.amjcard.2003.08.053] [PMID: 14675580]

[84]   Dokainish H, Zoghbi WA, Lakkis NM, Quinones MA, Nagueh SF. Comparative accuracy of B-type natriuretic peptide and tissue Doppler echocardiography in the diagnosis of congestive heart failure. Am J Cardiol 2004; 93(9): 1130-5.
[http://dx.doi.org/10.1016/j.amjcard.2004.01.042] [PMID: 15110205]

[85] Pinamonti B, Zecchin M, Di Lenarda A, Gregori D, Sinagra G, Camerini F. Persistence of restrictive left ventricular filling pattern in dilated cardiomyopathy: an ominous prognostic sign. J Am Coll Cardiol 1997; 29(3): 604-12.
[http://dx.doi.org/10.1016/S0735-1097(96)00539-6] [PMID: 9060900]

[86] Cohn JN, Ferrari R, Sharpe N. Cardiac remodeling--concepts and clinical implications: a consensus paper from an international forum on cardiac remodeling. Behalf of an International Forum on Cardiac Remodeling. J Am Coll Cardiol 2000; 35(3): 569-82.
[http://dx.doi.org/10.1016/S0735-1097(99)00630-0] [PMID: 10716457]

[87] Sutton MG, Sharpe N. Left ventricular remodeling after myocardial infarction: pathophysiology and therapy. Circulation 2000; 101(25): 2981-8.
[http://dx.doi.org/10.1161/01.CIR.101.25.2981] [PMID: 10869273]

[88] McKay RG, Pfeffer MA, Pasternak RC, et al. Left ventricular remodeling after myocardial infarction: a corollary to infarct expansion. Circulation 1986; 74(4): 693-702.
[http://dx.doi.org/10.1161/01.CIR.74.4.693] [PMID: 3757183]

[89] Rumberger JA, Behrenbeck T, Breen JR, Reed JE, Gersh BJ. Nonparallel changes in global left ventricular chamber volume and muscle mass during the first year after transmural myocardial infarction in humans. J Am Coll Cardiol 1993; 21(3): 673-82.
[http://dx.doi.org/10.1016/0735-1097(93)90100-F] [PMID: 8436749]

[90] St John Sutton M, Pfeffer MA, Plappert T, et al. Quantitative two-dimensional echocardiographic measurements are major predictors of adverse cardiovascular events after acute myocardial infarction. The protective effects of captopril. Circulation 1994; 89(1): 68-75.
[http://dx.doi.org/10.1161/01.CIR.89.1.68] [PMID: 8281697]

[91] Mannaerts HF, van der Heide JA, Kamp O, Stoel MG, Twisk J, Visser CA. Early identification of left ventricular remodelling after myocardial infarction, assessed by transthoracic 3D echocardiography. Eur Heart J 2004; 25(8): 680-7.
[http://dx.doi.org/10.1016/j.ehj.2004.02.030] [PMID: 15084373]

[92] Grossman W, Jones D, McLaurin LP. Wall stress and patterns of hypertrophy in the human left ventricle. J Clin Invest 1975; 56(1): 56-64.
[http://dx.doi.org/10.1172/JCI108079] [PMID: 124746]

[93] Ganau A, Devereux RB, Roman MJ, et al. Patterns of left ventricular hypertrophy and geometric remodeling in essential hypertension. J Am Coll Cardiol 1992; 19(7): 1550-8.
[http://dx.doi.org/10.1016/0735-1097(92)90617-V] [PMID: 1534335]

[94] Quiñones MA, Greenberg BH, Kopelen HA, et al. Echocardiographic predictors of clinical outcome in patients with left ventricular dysfunction enrolled in the SOLVD registry and trials: significance of left ventricular hypertrophy. Studies of Left Ventricular Dysfunction. J Am Coll Cardiol 2000; 35(5): 1237-44.
[http://dx.doi.org/10.1016/S0735-1097(00)00511-8] [PMID: 10758966]

[95] Tsang TS, Barnes ME, Bailey KR, et al. Left atrial volume: important risk marker of incident atrial fibrillation in 1655 older men and women. Mayo Clin Proc 2001; 76(5): 467-75.
[http://dx.doi.org/10.4065/76.5.467] [PMID: 11357793]

[96] Rossi A, Cicoira M, Zanolla L, et al. Determinants and prognostic value of left atrial volume in patients with dilated cardiomyopathy. J Am Coll Cardiol 2002; 40(8): 1425.
[http://dx.doi.org/10.1016/S0735-1097(02)02305-7] [PMID: 12392832]

[97] Teerlink JR, Goldhaber SZ, Pfeffer MA. An overview of contemporary etiologies of congestive heart failure. Am Heart J 1991; 121(6 Pt 1): 1852-3.
[http://dx.doi.org/10.1016/0002-8703(91)90072-P] [PMID: 2035416]

[98] Schulz R, Heusch G. Characterization of hibernating and stunned myocardium Eur Heart J 1995; 16 (J): 19-25.

[http://dx.doi.org/10.1093/eurheartj/16.suppl_J.19]

[99]   Beckmann S, *et al.* Diagnosis of coronary artery disease and viable myocardium by stress echocardiography Diagnostic accuracy of different stress modalities Eur Heart J 1995; 16 (J): 10-8.
[http://dx.doi.org/10.1093/eurheartj/16.suppl_J.10]

[100] Picano E. Stress echocardiography. From pathophysiological toy to diagnostic tool. Circulation 1992; 85(4): 1604-12.
[http://dx.doi.org/10.1161/01.CIR.85.4.1604] [PMID: 1555297]

[101] Nagueh SF, Mikati I, Weilbaecher D, *et al.* Relation of the contractile reserve of hibernating myocardium to myocardial structure in humans. Circulation 1999; 100(5): 490-6.
[http://dx.doi.org/10.1161/01.CIR.100.5.490] [PMID: 10430762]

[102] Baer FM, Voth E, Deutsch HJ, *et al.* Predictive value of low dose dobutamine transesophageal echocardiography and fluorine-18 fluorodeoxyglucose positron emission tomography for recovery of regional left ventricular function after successful revascularization. J Am Coll Cardiol 1996; 28(1): 60-9.
[http://dx.doi.org/10.1016/0735-1097(96)00106-4] [PMID: 8752795]

[103] Senior R, Lahiri A. Role of dobutamine echocardiography in detection of myocardial viability for predicting outcome after revascularization in ischemic cardiomyopathy. J Am Soc Echocardiogr 2001; 14(3): 240-8.
[http://dx.doi.org/10.1067/mje.2001.107636] [PMID: 11241023]

[104] Pratali L, Picano E, Otasevic P, *et al.* Prognostic significance of the dobutamine echocardiography test in idiopathic dilated cardiomyopathy. Am J Cardiol 2001; 88(12): 1374-8.
[http://dx.doi.org/10.1016/S0002-9149(01)02116-6] [PMID: 11741555]

[105] Matsumoto K, Tanaka H, Onishi A, *et al.* Bi-ventricular contractile reserve offers an incremental prognostic value for patients with dilated cardiomyopathy. Eur Heart J Cardiovasc Imaging 2015; 16(11): 1213-23.
[http://dx.doi.org/10.1093/ehjci/jev069] [PMID: 25851330]

[106] Nagueh SF, Appleton CP, Gillebert TC, *et al.* Recommendations for the evaluation of left ventricular diastolic function by echocardiography. Eur J Echocardiogr 2009; 10(2): 165-93.
[http://dx.doi.org/10.1093/ejechocard/jep007] [PMID: 19270053]

[107] Polak JF, Holman BL, Wynne J, Colucci WS. Right ventricular ejection fraction: an indicator of increased mortality in patients with congestive heart failure associated with coronary artery disease. J Am Coll Cardiol 1983; 2(2): 217-24.
[http://dx.doi.org/10.1016/S0735-1097(83)80156-9] [PMID: 6306086]

[108] Gavazzi A, Berzuini C, Campana C, *et al.* Value of right ventricular ejection fraction in predicting short-term prognosis of patients with severe chronic heart failure. J Heart Lung Transplant 1997; 16(7): 774-85.
[PMID: 9257260]

[109] de Groote P, Millaire A, Foucher-Hossein C, *et al.* Right ventricular ejection fraction is an independent predictor of survival in patients with moderate heart failure. J Am Coll Cardiol 1998; 32(4): 948-54.
[http://dx.doi.org/10.1016/S0735-1097(98)00337-4] [PMID: 9768716]

[110] Kaul S, Tei C, Hopkins JM, Shah PM. Assessment of right ventricular function using two-dimensional echocardiography. Am Heart J 1984; 107(3): 526-31.
[http://dx.doi.org/10.1016/0002-8703(84)90095-4] [PMID: 6695697]

[111] Lindqvist P, Waldenström A, Henein M, Mörner S, Kazzam E. Regional and global right ventricular function in healthy individuals aged 20-90 years: a pulsed Doppler tissue imaging study: Umeå General Population Heart Study. Echocardiography 2005; 22(4): 305-14.
[http://dx.doi.org/10.1111/j.1540-8175.2005.04023.x] [PMID: 15839985]

[112] Lai WW, Gauvreau K, Rivera ES, Saleeb S, Powell AJ, Geva T. Accuracy of guideline recommendations for two-dimensional quantification of the right ventricle by echocardiography. Int J Cardiovasc Imaging 2008; 24(7): 691-8.
[http://dx.doi.org/10.1007/s10554-008-9314-4] [PMID: 18438737]

[113] Nass N, *et al.* Recovery of regional right ventricular function after thrombolysis for pulmonary embolism Am J Cardiol 1999; 83(5): 804-6. A10
[http://dx.doi.org/10.1016/S0002-9149(98)01000-5]

[114] Zornoff LA, Skali H, Pfeffer MA, *et al.* Right ventricular dysfunction and risk of heart failure and mortality after myocardial infarction. J Am Coll Cardiol 2002; 39(9): 1450-5.
[http://dx.doi.org/10.1016/S0735-1097(02)01804-1] [PMID: 11985906]

[115] Anavekar NS, Skali H, Bourgoun M, *et al.* Usefulness of right ventricular fractional area change to predict death, heart failure, and stroke following myocardial infarction (from the VALIANT ECHO Study). Am J Cardiol 2008; 101(5): 607-12.
[http://dx.doi.org/10.1016/j.amjcard.2007.09.115] [PMID: 18308007]

[116] Abd El Rahman MY, Abdul-Khaliq H, Vogel M, *et al.* Value of the new Doppler-derived myocardial performance index for the evaluation of right and left ventricular function following repair of tetralogy of fallot. Pediatr Cardiol 2002; 23(5): 502-7.
[http://dx.doi.org/10.1007/s00246-002-1469-5] [PMID: 12189405]

[117] Chockalingam A, Gnanavelu G, Alagesan R, Subramaniam T. Myocardial performance index in evaluation of acute right ventricular myocardial infarction. Echocardiography 2004; 21(6): 487-94.
[http://dx.doi.org/10.1111/j.0742-2822.2004.03139.x] [PMID: 15298683]

[118] Eidem BW, O'Leary PW, Tei C, Seward JB. Usefulness of the myocardial performance index for assessing right ventricular function in congenital heart disease. Am J Cardiol 2000; 86(6): 654-8.
[http://dx.doi.org/10.1016/S0002-9149(00)01047-X] [PMID: 10980218]

[119] Mörner S, Lindqvist P, Waldenström A, Kazzam E. Right ventricular dysfunction in hypertrophic cardiomyopathy as evidenced by the myocardial performance index. Int J Cardiol 2008; 124(1): 57-63.
[http://dx.doi.org/10.1016/j.ijcard.2006.12.022] [PMID: 17383757]

[120] Motoki H, Borowski AG, Shrestha K, *et al.* Right ventricular global longitudinal strain provides prognostic value incremental to left ventricular ejection fraction in patients with heart failure. J Am Soc Echocardiogr 2014; 27(7): 726-32.
[http://dx.doi.org/10.1016/j.echo.2014.02.007] [PMID: 24679740]

[121] Felker GM, Thompson RE, Hare JM, *et al.* Underlying causes and long-term survival in patients with initially unexplained cardiomyopathy. N Engl J Med 2000; 342(15): 1077-84.
[http://dx.doi.org/10.1056/NEJM200004133421502] [PMID: 10760308]

[122] Baumgartner H, Hung J, Bermejo J, *et al.* Echocardiographic assessment of valve stenosis: EAE/ASE recommendations for clinical practice. Eur J Echocardiogr 2009; 10(1): 1-25.
[http://dx.doi.org/10.1093/ejechocard/jen303] [PMID: 19065003]

[123] Nesta F, Otsuji Y, Handschumacher MD, *et al.* Leaflet concavity: a rapid visual clue to the presence and mechanism of functional mitral regurgitation. J Am Soc Echocardiogr 2003; 16(12): 1301-8.
[http://dx.doi.org/10.1067/j.echo.2003.09.003] [PMID: 14652610]

[124] Kwan J, Shiota T, Agler DA, *et al.* Geometric differences of the mitral apparatus between ischemic and dilated cardiomyopathy with significant mitral regurgitation: real-time three-dimensional echocardiography study. Circulation 2003; 107(8): 1135-40.
[http://dx.doi.org/10.1161/01.CIR.0000053558.55471.2D] [PMID: 12615791]

[125] Yared K, Baggish AL, Picard MH, Hoffmann U, Hung J. Multimodality imaging of pericardial diseases. JACC Cardiovasc Imaging 2010; 3(6): 650-60.
[http://dx.doi.org/10.1016/j.jcmg.2010.04.009] [PMID: 20541720]

[126] Dal-Bianco JP, Sengupta PP, Mookadam F, Chandrasekaran K, Tajik AJ, Khandheria BK. Role of

echocardiography in the diagnosis of constrictive pericarditis. J Am Soc Echocardiogr 2009; 22(1): 24-33.
[http://dx.doi.org/10.1016/j.echo.2008.11.004] [PMID: 19130999]

[127] Randomised, placebo-controlled trial of carvedilol in patients with congestive heart failure due to ischaemic heart disease. Lancet 1997; 349(9049): 375-80.
[http://dx.doi.org/10.1016/S0140-6736(97)80008-6] [PMID: 9033462]

[128] Tassan-Mangina S, Codorean D, Metivier M, *et al.* Tissue Doppler imaging and conventional echocardiography after anthracycline treatment in adults: early and late alterations of left ventricular function during a prospective study. Eur J Echocardiogr 2006; 7(2): 141-6.
[http://dx.doi.org/10.1016/j.euje.2005.04.009] [PMID: 15941672]

[129] Francis GS. Development of arrhythmias in the patient with congestive heart failure: pathophysiology, prevalence and prognosis. Am J Cardiol 1986; 57(3): 3B-7B.
[http://dx.doi.org/10.1016/0002-9149(86)90991-4] [PMID: 3946204]

[130] Holmes J, Kubo SH, Cody RJ, Kligfield P. Arrhythmias in ischemic and nonischemic dilated cardiomyopathy: prediction of mortality by ambulatory electrocardiography. Am J Cardiol 1985; 55(1): 146-51.
[http://dx.doi.org/10.1016/0002-9149(85)90317-0] [PMID: 3881000]

[131] Moss AJ, Hall WJ, Cannom DS, *et al.* Improved survival with an implanted defibrillator in patients with coronary disease at high risk for ventricular arrhythmia. N Engl J Med 1996; 335(26): 1933-40.
[http://dx.doi.org/10.1056/NEJM199612263352601] [PMID: 8960472]

[132] Moss AJ, Zareba W, Hall WJ, *et al.* Prophylactic implantation of a defibrillator in patients with myocardial infarction and reduced ejection fraction. N Engl J Med 2002; 346(12): 877-83.
[http://dx.doi.org/10.1056/NEJMoa013474] [PMID: 11907286]

[133] Bardy GH, Lee KL, Mark DB, *et al.* Amiodarone or an implantable cardioverter-defibrillator for congestive heart failure. N Engl J Med 2005; 352(3): 225-37.
[http://dx.doi.org/10.1056/NEJMoa043399] [PMID: 15659722]

[134] Leclercq C, Kass DA. Retiming the failing heart: principles and current clinical status of cardiac resynchronization. J Am Coll Cardiol 2002; 39(2): 194-201.
[http://dx.doi.org/10.1016/S0735-1097(01)01747-8] [PMID: 11788207]

[135] Bristow MR, Saxon LA, Boehmer J, *et al.* Cardiac-resynchronization therapy with or without an implantable defibrillator in advanced chronic heart failure. N Engl J Med 2004; 350(21): 2140-50.
[http://dx.doi.org/10.1056/NEJMoa032423] [PMID: 15152059]

[136] Cleland JG, Daubert JC, Erdmann E, *et al.* The effect of cardiac resynchronization on morbidity and mortality in heart failure. N Engl J Med 2005; 352(15): 1539-49.
[http://dx.doi.org/10.1056/NEJMoa050496] [PMID: 15753115]

[137] St John Sutton MG, Plappert T, Abraham WT, *et al.* Effect of cardiac resynchronization therapy on left ventricular size and function in chronic heart failure. Circulation 2003; 107(15): 1985-90.
[http://dx.doi.org/10.1161/01.CIR.0000065226.24159.E9] [PMID: 12668512]

[138] Breithardt OA, Sinha AM, Schwammenthal E, *et al.* Acute effects of cardiac resynchronization therapy on functional mitral regurgitation in advanced systolic heart failure. J Am Coll Cardiol 2003; 41(5): 765-70.
[http://dx.doi.org/10.1016/S0735-1097(02)02937-6] [PMID: 12628720]

[139] Russo AM, Stainback RF, Bailey SR, *et al.* ACCF/HRS/AHA/ASE/HFSA/SCAI/SCCT/SCMR 2013 appropriate use criteria for implantable cardioverter-defibrillators and cardiac resynchronization therapy: a report of the American College of Cardiology Foundation appropriate use criteria task force, Heart Rhythm Society, American Heart Association, American Society of Echocardiography, Heart Failure Society of America, Society for Cardiovascular Angiography and Interventions, Society of Cardiovascular Computed Tomography, and Society for Cardiovascular Magnetic Resonance. J Am Coll Cardiol 2013; 61(12): 1318-68.

[http://dx.doi.org/10.1016/j.jacc.2012.12.017] [PMID: 23453819]

[140] Khan FZ, Virdee MS, Palmer CR, *et al.* Targeted left ventricular lead placement to guide cardiac resynchronization therapy: the TARGET study: a randomized, controlled trial. J Am Coll Cardiol 2012; 59(17): 1509-18.
[http://dx.doi.org/10.1016/j.jacc.2011.12.030] [PMID: 22405632]

[141] Saba S, Marek J, Schwartzman D, *et al.* Echocardiography-guided left ventricular lead placement for cardiac resynchronization therapy: results of the Speckle Tracking Assisted Resynchronization Therapy for Electrode Region trial. Circ Heart Fail 2013; 6(3): 427-34.
[http://dx.doi.org/10.1161/CIRCHEARTFAILURE.112.000078] [PMID: 23476053]

[142] Park JH, Negishi K, Grimm RA, *et al.* Echocardiographic predictors of reverse remodeling after cardiac resynchronization therapy and subsequent events. Circ Cardiovasc Imaging 2013; 6(6): 864-72.
[http://dx.doi.org/10.1161/CIRCIMAGING.112.000026] [PMID: 24084489]

[143] Cleveland JC Jr, Naftel DC, Reece TB, *et al.* Survival after biventricular assist device implantation: an analysis of the Interagency Registry for Mechanically Assisted Circulatory Support database. J Heart Lung Transplant 2011; 30(8): 862-9.
[http://dx.doi.org/10.1016/j.healun.2011.04.004] [PMID: 21621423]

[144] Todaro MC, Khandheria BK, Paterick TE, Umland MM, Thohan V. The practical role of echocardiography in selection, implantation, and management of patients requiring LVAD therapy. Curr Cardiol Rep 2014; 16(4): 468.
[http://dx.doi.org/10.1007/s11886-014-0468-5] [PMID: 24585110]

[145] Grant AD, Smedira NG, Starling RC, Marwick TH. Independent and incremental role of quantitative right ventricular evaluation for the prediction of right ventricular failure after left ventricular assist device implantation. J Am Coll Cardiol 2012; 60(6): 521-8.
[http://dx.doi.org/10.1016/j.jacc.2012.02.073] [PMID: 22858287]

[146] Shapiro GC, Leibowitz DW, Oz MC, Weslow RG, Di Tullio MR, Homma S. Diagnosis of patent foramen ovale with transesophageal echocardiography in a patient supported with a left ventricular assist device. J Heart Lung Transplant 1995; 14(3): 594-7.
[PMID: 7654743]

[147] Reilly MP, *et al.* Frequency, risk factors, and clinical outcomes of left ventricular assist device-associated ventricular thrombus Am J Cardiol 2000; 86(10): 1156-9. A10
[http://dx.doi.org/10.1016/S0002-9149(00)01182-6]

[148] Horton SC, Khodaverdian R, Chatelain P, *et al.* Left ventricular assist device malfunction: an approach to diagnosis by echocardiography. J Am Coll Cardiol 2005; 45(9): 1435-40.
[http://dx.doi.org/10.1016/j.jacc.2005.01.037] [PMID: 15862415]

[149] Yancy CW, Jessup M, Bozkurt B, *et al.* 2013 ACCF/AHA guideline for the management of heart failure: executive summary: a report of the American College of Cardiology Foundation/American Heart Association Task Force on practice guidelines. Circulation 2013; 128(16): 1810-52.
[http://dx.doi.org/10.1161/CIR.0b013e31829e8807] [PMID: 23741057]

[150] Ammar KA, Jacobsen SJ, Mahoney DW, *et al.* Prevalence and prognostic significance of heart failure stages: application of the American College of Cardiology/American Heart Association heart failure staging criteria in the community. Circulation 2007; 115(12): 1563-70.
[http://dx.doi.org/10.1161/CIRCULATIONAHA.106.666818] [PMID: 17353436]

CHAPTER 5

Role of Cardiac Imaging in Heart Failure

Ahmed Aljizeeri[*], **Ahmed Alsaileek** and **Mouaz H. Al-Mallah**

King Abdulaziz Cardiac Center, King Abdulaziz Medical City-Riyadh, Riyadh, Kingdom of Saudi Arabia

Abstract: Non-invasive cardiac imaging plays a pivotal role in the contemporary care of heart failure. It has a tremendous potential for better comprehension of the mechanism of heart failure, detection of subclinical disease, assessment and classification of the current state of the established disease and provision of insights regarding prognosis and response to therapy. Cardiac magnetic resonance (CMR), cardiac computed tomography (CCT) and nuclear cardiology provide robust diagnostic and prognostic information. CMR provides the most comprehensive information but it is limited by the availability. Nuclear cardiology, particularly positron emission tomography (PET), provides high diagnostic yield and has exceptional potential in molecular imaging, but is limited by the ionizing radiation and availability. CCT has an established role in the diagnosis of coronary artery disease and an evolving role in tissue characterization, but like nuclear cardiology, it is limited by associated radiation exposure. This chapter discusses the role of CMR, CCT and nuclear cardiology in the management of heart failure.

Keywords: Cardiac Computed Tomography, Cardiac computed Tomography Angiography, Cardiomyopathy, Cardiovascular Mgnetic Resonance, Coronary Artery Disease, Myocardial Delayed Enhancement, Diastolic Dysfunction, Ejection Fraction, Gated SPECT, Heart Failure, Late Gadolinium Enhancement, Micro-Vascular Obstruction, Myocardial Function, Myocardial Innervation, Myocardial Perfusion, Myocardial Viability, Nuclear Cardiology, Positron Emission Tomography, Radionuclide Angiography, Single Photon Emission Tomography.

INTRODUCTION

Nowadays, cardiac imaging plays a pivotal role in the evaluation of patients with heart failure. It is used in the initial evaluation, diagnosis, prognostication and choice of medical and surgical therapy of heart failure. Its role has been consistently emphasized by the international scientific societies guidelines of

---

[*] **Corresponding author Ahmed Aljizeeri:** King Abdulaziz Cardiac Center, King Abdulaziz Medical City-Riyadh, Riyadh, Kingdom of Saudi Arabia; Tel: +966 11 8011111; Ext: 10485; E-mail: aljizeeri@yahoo.com

Mohammad El Tahlawi (Ed.)
All rights reserved-© 2020 Bentham Science Publishers

heart failure management [1, 2]. Moreover, the role of cardiac imaging is expected to increase with the current epidemic of heart failure as a result of aging population and recent advances and improvement in the care of coronary artery disease [3, 4]. 2-Dimensional echocardiography remains the first diagnostic modality for the assessment of heart failure. However, the acoustic window, geometric assumption in quantification of the left ventricular ejection fraction and inability to detect minute changes in ejection fraction are known limitations of echocardiography that are not seen in other imaging modalities. This chapter discusses the role of cardiovascular magnetic resonance (CMR), Cardiovascular Computed Tomography (CCT) and Nuclear Scintigraphy in the management of patients with heart failure and reduced as well as preserved ejection fraction.

CARDIOVASCULAR MAGNETIC RESONANCE IMAGING

In recent years, Cardiovascular Magnetic Resonance (CMR) has emerged as an important tool in the evaluation and quantification of ventricular size and function, and myocardial viability in heart failure. The precise quantification, nonuse of ionized radiation and the ability for tissue characterization give CMR a superior role over the other imaging modality.

CMR Techniques and Protocols

CMR has a wide range of clinical applications in contemporary cardiac care. It has an established role in the anatomical evaluation of various cardiac structures, including cardiac chambers, valves, pericardium and major vessels. It can help in the assessment of ventricular function and detection of ischemic heart disease [5, 6].

Different forms of protocols are employed to obtain image sequences to evaluate different components of the heart. Frequently used sequences include cine images to evaluate the size and function of the ventricles as well as wall motion, edema images to evaluate the presence of myocardial edema which usually denotes an acute process and delayed enhancement images to evaluate myocardial injury [7]. A T2* image is a sequence that evaluates the local magnetic field inhomogeneity that results from iron deposition within the myocardium seen in certain cardiomyopathies. The delayed enhancement images are obtained after administration of an intravenous gadolinium-based contrast agent (GBCA) [8]. CMR stress myocardial perfusion can be performed with either dobutamine or a vasodilator agent during which GBCA is injected at peak stress or hyperemia [7]. GDBA is also used for magnetic resonance angiography, although its role in coronary angiography is limited [9]. Flow quantification sequences are used to evaluate and grade the severity of valvular regurgitation [10, 11].

Although CMR exam utilizes the properties of the nuclei, it does not alter its structure since it does not involve the use of ionizing radiation. Therefore, the use of CMR can be performed repeatedly even at a young age without the risk of future development of malignancy. Moreover, the GBCA does not affect the kidney function; however, GBCA is contraindicated in patient with severe renal dysfunction (glomerular filtration rate < 30 ml/min/1.73 m^2) or patients on heamodialysis due to possibility of developing Nephrogenic Systemic Fibrosis (NSF), a rare and serious condition characterized by fibrosis of the skin, eye and joint following exposure to GBCA [12]. Finally, care should be taken while performing CMR in patients with pacemaker and automated implantable cardiac defibrillator (AICD). The magnetic field may cause heating of the implanted leads or may result in alteration of the programming of these devices [13]. Newer devices, however, are CMR compatible and therefore, allow performing the CMR study with some precautions [14].

Heart Failure with Reduced Ejection Fraction

Heart failure is a clinical syndrome that manifests irrespective of left ventricular ejection fraction (LVEF). Two clinical entities have been described in heart failure patients; heart failure with reduced ejection fraction (HFrEF), LVEF ≤ 40% also known and systolic dysfunction and heart failure with preserved ejection fraction (HFpEF), LVEF ≥50% also known and diastolic heart failure (1). Quantification of LVEF is essential in the proper classification and prognostication of HF patients [15]. In fact, precise quantification of LVEF is crucial in clinical decision making in regards to medical and device therapy in patients with HFrEF [16, 17]. Two-dimensional echocardiography (2D echo) is conventionally used in the estimation of LVEF. However, 2D echo has its limitation in evaluation of the LVEF including geometric assumption, inter-observer variability in addition to inherent limitation of poor acoustic window in some patients [18, 19]. CMR has emerged as an accurate alternative to overcome these shortcomings.

CMR and Quantification of Ventricular Volumes and Systolic Function

The high spatial resolution, excellent endocardial border definition and ability to image the heart in multiple planes give CMR superiority over other imaging modalities in the evaluation of ventricular volumes and systolic function [20]. Additionally, CMR allows for volumetric assessment independent of geometric assumptions even in patients with substantial remodeling [21, 22]. This is particularly important in the evaluation right ventricle (RV) due to its complex 3-dimentional and highly variable morphology. Hence, CMR evaluation is very accurate and highly reproducible irrespective of body habitus, ventricular remodeling or the degree of systolic dysfunction [23, 24]. Equivalently, the delineation of endocardial borders allows for accurate identification of wall motion abnormalities [25]. Currently, CMR is considered the gold standard method for evaluating both the left (LV) and the right ventricular (RV) size and systolic function [21, 26].

CMR plays an important role in the management of patients with heart failure by providing accurate quantification and detecting changes of LVEF. LVEF is the most important parameter for the choice of medical and device therapy in heart failure. Addition of aldosterone antagonist should be considered heart failure patients with New York Heart Association (NYHA) class II-IV and LVEF $\leq 35\%$ (1). Similarly, LVEF dictates the need for cardiac resynchronization therapy [27]. It is also a strong and independent predictor of arrhythmic death in patients with heart failure. Prophylactic implantation of AICD is indicated for primary prevention in patients with reduced LVEF who have received maximal medical therapy [1, 27]. Left ventricular (LV) dilatation has also been identified as a measure of poor prognosis in patients with heart failure [28]. Right ventricular (RV) size and ejection fraction are also parameters of poor prognosis in heart failure [29 - 31]. In patients with myocardial infarction, RVEF has been shown to have prognostic value independent of infarct size and LVEF [32].

CMR and the Diagnosis of Early Stage Heart Failure

The diagnosis of early stages of heart failure (stage A and B) is crucial for the initiation of therapy and to prevent the progression of the disease. CMR provides accurate and precise quantification of LVEF and LV mass and therefore allows for detection of early stages of heart failure and subsequent initiation of appropriate therapy. Moreover, tissue characterizations with CMR techniques like T2* help early identification of disease process such as cardiac iron overload in thalassemia patients and thereby helps preventing the progression of the disease into overt heart failure.

CMR and the Etiology of Heat Failure with Reduced Ejection Fraction

HFrEF can be caused by many pathologies including coronary artery disease (CAD), hypertension (HTN), valvular heart disease, myocarditis, HIV, toxin such as alcohol and cancer chemotherapy as well as idiopathic dilated cardiomyopathy (DCM) [33]. CAD remains the most common cause of heart failure [34, 35] and carries the worst prognosis [36, 37]. CAD is traditionally diagnosed by invasive coronary angiography (ICA). However, invasive coronary angiography may not be necessary in patients with heart failure and low likelihood of having CAD. Scientific societies recommend non-invasive stress testing before ICA in this group of patients. Recently, CMR has emerged as an alternative modality to detect CAD as an etiology of heart failure through myocardial tissue characterization by myocardial delayed enhancement.

Myocardial delayed enhancement (MDE) or late gadolinium enhancement (LGE) is a CMR imaging sequence utilized for myocardial tissue characterization. It allows for identification of the etiology of heart failure and also helps in differentiating stunned from nonviable myocardium in ischemic heart failure. Gadolinium is an extracellular contrast agent that does not cross intact cell membrane. However, cellular damage, during acute myocardial infarction (MI) and in case of increase in the extracellular fibrosis in chronic MI, increases the distribution volume of gadolinium [38, 39]. Moreover, there is a delayed washout of gadolinium contrast from damaged myocardium in comparison to normal myocardium [40]. Therefore, obtaining CMR images 10-15 minutes after intravenous administration of GBCA permits the differentiation between normal and abnormal myocardium. The abnormal myocardium appears as white, hyperenhanced, while normal myocardium appears as black because gadolinium has completely washed out from normal myocardium. The location, pattern and extent of MDE provide valuable diagnostic and prognostic information [41 - 44].

Ischemic Delayed Myocardial Enhancement

Ischemic cardiomyopathy (ICM) has a typical pattern of MDE characterized by areas of fibrosis seen in the subendocardium of a coronary artery territory that may extend into the epicardium depending on the transmurality of the infarct [43, 45] (Fig. **1**). The extent of the MDE within thickness of the myocardial segment is a measure of viability and has been shown to predict functional recovery after revascularization. Involvement of less than 25% of the thickness of the segment is associated with high likelihood of recovery, while involvement of more than 75% portends a low likelihood of recovery [46 - 48]. The addition of CMR edema imaging (T2-weighted images) to MDE can help differentiate acute from chronic myocardial injury as edema is only seen during the acute process [49]. Furthermore, quantification of edema and fibrosis can help in identification of salvaged myocardium that is represented by the area of edema and no MDE [50]. The peri-infarct zone has also been shown to predict future arrhythmia [51, 52]. The presence of edema can also help in detecting areas that had ischemia with no infarction [53, 54]. On the other hand, the high spatial resolution of CMR permits recognition of small subendocardial infarctions that can be missed by other imaging modalities and are prognostically important [55]. The ischemic MDE has high sensitivity of detecting CAD [41]. However, 15% of patients with ICM has no or non-ischemic DE, which can be due to presence of collaterals, hibernation or concomitant non-ischemic process [56, 57]. In addition, approximately 13% of patients with non-obstructive CAD have MDE that resembles CAD and may be related to recanalization of the culprit artery, vasospasm or embolic phenomenon [41].

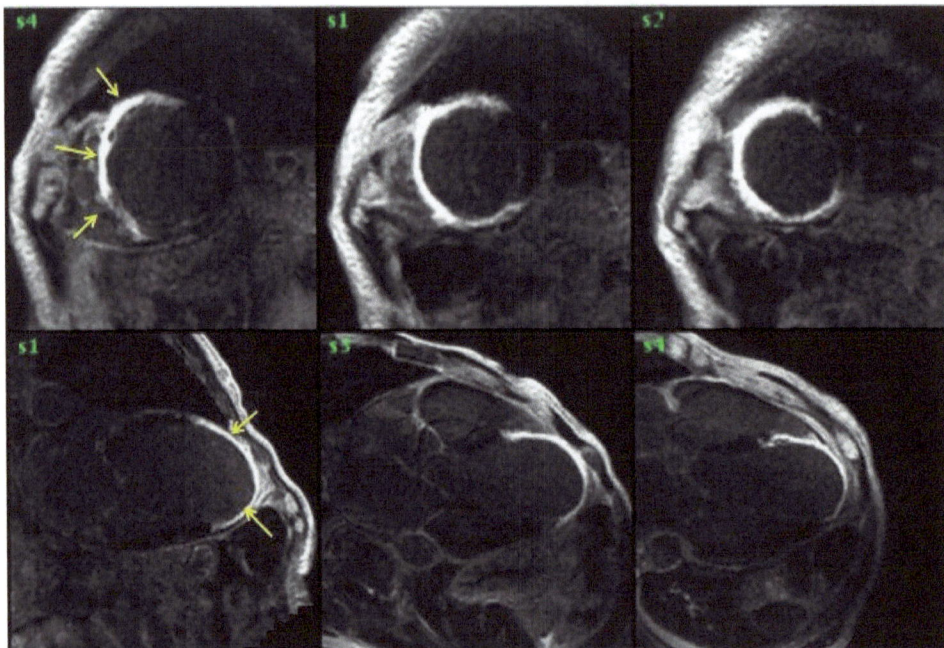

Fig. (1). Delayed myocardial enhancement image showing transmural myocardial delayed enhancement in the anterior and anteroseptal wall (LAD *territory*) (*yellow arrows*) indicating ischemic cause in a patient presenting with new onset heart failure.

Administration of GBCA can also help in detection of other complication of MI. Microvascular obstruction (MVO) results from failure of microvascular perfusion despite restoration of epicardial coronary flow. This could be either due to capillary occlusion by microthrmbi [58]. MVO has been recognized as a strong predicator of LV remodeling independent of extent of infarction [59, 60] and is associated with increased major cardiac events including cardiac death, nonfatal MI, hospitalization for heart failure and ischemic stroke [61]. Addition of T2* imaging can identify intra-myocardial hemorrhage that can complicate MVO in the setting of acute MI. Like MVO, intramyocardial hemorrhage was shown to be a predictor of adverse LV remodeling independent of infarct size [62].

Finally, CMR helps in detection of other complications of CAD, including LV aneurysms, LV thrombi and papillary muscle infarction. CMR is superior to other imaging modalities in detecting thrombi and evaluation of LV aneurysms due to its high spatial resolution and ability to image in 3-diemential planes [63 - 66].

Therefore, the combination of cine images, edema images, T2* and MDE images provides CMR with the ability to identify all the pathophysiological processes involved in the development of heart failure in CAD including myocardial scar, stunning, hibernation and LV remodeling. On the other hand, it provides therapeutic and prognostic insights into the management of such patients.

Ischemia Evaluation- Stress CMR Perfusion

Assessment of CAD is a cornerstone in initial workup for HFrEF. In recent years, CMR has evolved to be an accurate modality in detecting ischemia in patients with suspected CAD. Vasodilator stress CMR has a sensitivity and specificity of 91% and 83% in comparison to ICA, respectively [67]. Stress CMR performs better than single-photon emission tomography in detecting ischemia both in male and females [68]. Several studies have shown the feasibility and safety of CMR stress perfusion with either vasodilator or dobutamine [69 - 71]. The visualization of wall motion abnormalities with dobutamine improves the diagnostic accuracy of stress CMR and can help in quantification of contractile reserve. This can also help in evaluating the possible recovery of segments with intermediate MDE [72]. The high diagnostic accuracy and lack of ionizing radiation make CMR stress perfusion a preferred test especially in women and young patients. The most recent guidelines, European Society of Cardiology, recommend stress CMR as an initial step in the workup of heart failure with suspected CAD [2, 73].

CMR Coronary Angiography

Although recent studies have demonstrated reasonable diagnostic ability of CMR coronary angiography in detecting > 50% stenosis in proximal and mid coronary artery segments [74, 75], its routine clinical use is limited by the small size of the coronary artery, motion artifact and operator expertise. For those reasons, scientific societies limited their recommendation of CMR coronary angiography to the evaluation of coronary artery anomalies [76].

Non-ischemic Delayed Myocardial Enhancement Cardiomyopathy

Dilated Cardiomyopathy

DCM has several etiologies some of which are reversible; however, most cases of DCM are idiopathic (50%) and less than 10% are due to CAD [33]. Around half of the patients with DCM have a familial type [77] and therefore early identification of these patients and screening their family members is essential in the management of DCM.

The diagnosis of DCM is typically made after exclusion of CAD. However, ICA may not be sufficient to entirely exclude ICM as some of the patients with heart failure were found to have ischemic MDE despite the absence of obstructive CAD on ICA, indicating possible ischemic etiology of HF [57]. The presence of ischemic MDE in this group of patients is thought be related to recanalization of the culprit artery, vasospasm or embolic phenomenon. Unlike ICM, DCM tends to have either no evidence of MDE (59% of cases) or mid wall patchy or longitudinal striae (28%) (Fig. **2**) [41]. Typically the areas of MDE do not correspond to a particular coronary artery territory but correlate well to areas of fibrosis on autopsy [78]. Hence, CMR can accurately differentiate between ischemic and non-ischemic cardiomyopathy without the need of invasive coronary angiography. This is particularly useful in patients with heart failure with low likelihood of CAD.

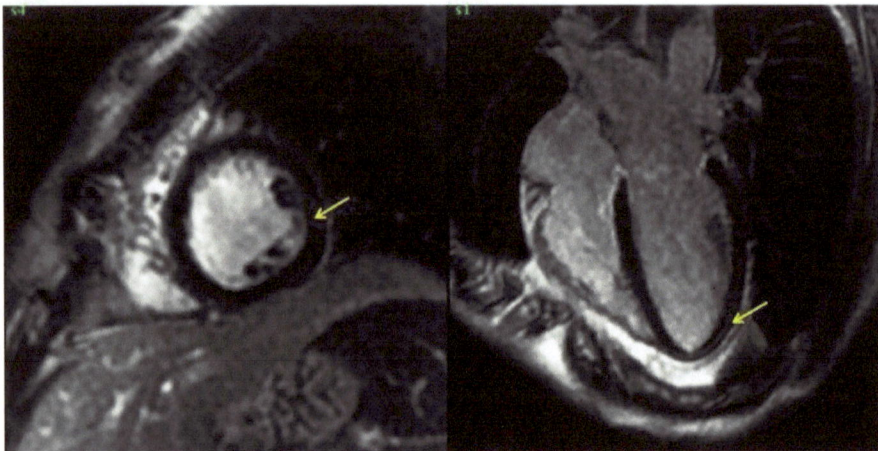

Fig. (2). Delayed myocardial enhancement image showing midwall delayed myocardial enhancement (*yellow arrows*) in a patient with dilated cardiomyopathy.

In addition to its diagnostic value, MDE provides incremental prognostic value in patients with cardiomyopathy to predict arrhythmias, sudden cardiac death, heart failure hospitalizations, future cardiac transplantation [79 - 81] as well as all-cause and cardiac mortality [82]. In addition, MDE is associated with an 8-fold increase in HF hospitalization, ICD discharges and cardiac death even after adjustment for LV volumes and EF [83].

Myocarditis

Viral myocarditis may result in long-term heart failure. Nearly 9% of DCM is caused by myocarditis [33]. Recently, The Lake Louise Criteria have been proposed to guide CMR diagnosis of myocarditis [84]. Based on these criteria, diagnosis of acute myocarditis is made if two out of three criteria are met, edema by T2-weighted images, hyperemia by early T1-weighted images and the presence of non-ischemic MDE. The MDE enhancement in myocarditis tends to affect the lateral and inferolateral wall and typically has a subepicardial distribution [85, 86] (Fig. **3**). In some cases of myocarditis, the MDE has a midwall distribution that resembles pattern seen in DCM, which supports the notion that some DCM cases are a sequel of myocarditis. Moreover, CMR can guide the endomyocardial biopsy and thus can improve its diagnostic yield [87].

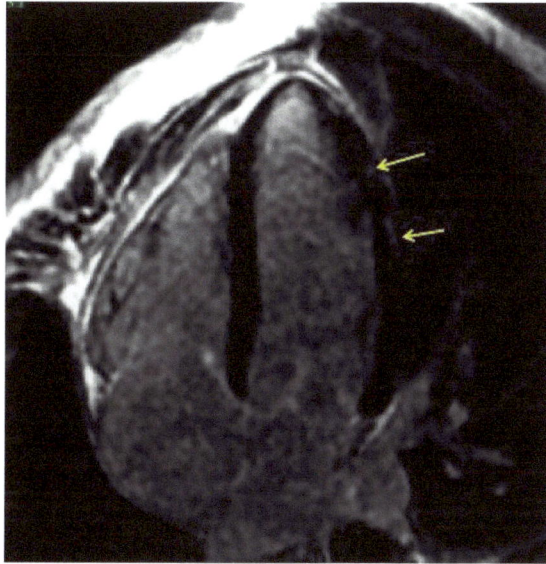

Fig. (3). Delayed myocardial enhancement image showing subepicardial delayed enhancement (*yellow arrows*) in a patient with myocarditis.

LV non-compaction Cardiomyopathy

Isolated LV non-compaction (LVNC) is a rare form of cardiomyopathy. The condition characterized by prominent LV trabeculations and the presence of inter-trabecular recesses [88]. The myocardium appears consisting of two layers, a thin compacted layer and a thick non-compacted layer. The diagnosis is made on echocardiography when the non-compacted/ compacted layer ratio is more than 2 in addition to the presence of deep myocardial recesses [89]. However, due to its limited spatial resolution, echocardiography can miss or overdiagnose some cases [90] particularly those with borderline abnormality or prior hypertensive heart disease. The high spatial resolution of CMR improves the diastolic accuracy allowing for better detection and measurement of the trabeculations. Similar to echocardiography, multiple CMR diagnostic criteria have been proposed [91]. These include a ratio of maximal non-compacted/compacted myocardium of more than 2.3 in end-diastole [92, 93] or a trabeculated LV mass more than 20% of global LV mass [94]. In LVNC, MDE is heterogeneous and correlates to the degree of LVEF [95, 96]. Additionally, CMR can detect concomitant prominent trabeculations of the RV associated with increased adverse clinical outcomes [97].

Cardiac Sarcoidosis

Cardiac sarcoidosis is an underdiagnosed condition characterized by heart failure, heart block or sudden cardiac dearth due to arrhythmia [98, 99]. Cardiac involvement can be seen in up to 25% of patient with sarcoidosis [100]. CMR or cardiac PET have been recently used in the evaluation of possible cardiac sarcoidosis. CMR provides information about the wall motion abnormalities, inflammation and fibrosis [101]. Increased T2-wieghted signal suggests edema which denotes active inflammation [102], while MDE reflects fibrosis. The MDE in sarcoidosis is typically patchy affecting the midwall mostly in the basal anteroseptal and inferolateral walls [103, 104] with frequent involvement of the papillary muscle [99]. MDE can also seen in the RV [105]. CMR is a part of the modified criteria of the Japanese Ministry of Heath for the diagnosis of cardiac sarcoidosis [106]. The presence of MDE in patients with cardiac sarcoidosis is associated with more than ten-fold increase in the risk of sudden cardiac death and nine-fold increase in clinical adverse events including appropriate AICD discharge and bradycardia requiring pacemaker insertion [107]. CMR can also be used to monitor response to disease modifying therapy by evaluation of progression of edema and MDE [108].

Iron Overload Cardiomyopathy

Iron overload cardiomyopathy is a secondary cardiomyopathy caused by excessive iron deposition in the myocardium secondary to frequent transfusions in hemoglobin disorders or abnormalities in iron metabolism [109]. As the myocardial iron increases, the LVEF decreases resulting in heart failure. CMR is increasingly used to evaluate patients with hemoglobinopathies and possible iron overload. $T2^*$ relaxation is primarily affected by hemosiderin and not by ferritin or cellular iron and therefore can be used to measure total myocardial iron deposition [110]. $T2^*$ relaxation time can be measured in full myocardial thickness or in the interventricular septum. In patients with thalassemia, a $T2^*$ value of less than 20 ms has been associated with iron overload and lower LVEF [111, 112], a value of less than 10 ms is associated with increased risk of heart failure and a value of less than 6 ms carries a high risk of arrhythmia [113]. Implementation of CMR-$T2^*$ in the follow up and guiding chelating agent therapy in patients with thalassemia has dramatically improved the survival of these patients. In UK (thalassemia registry) all-cause mortality has dropped from 12.7

to 4.3 per 1000 patient years after introduction of T2* in follow up of patients with thalassemia [114].

Stress (Tako-Tsubo) Cardiomyopathy

Stress (Tako-Tsubo) Cardiomyopathy is a reversible condition that mimics myocardial infarction and characterized by systolic dysfunction of the apical and mid segments of the LV without CAD [115, 116]. Stress cardiomyopathy features on CMR include a typical pattern of LV dysfunction of apical akinesis and ballooning, myocardial edema (T2-weighted) and the absence of significant necrosis/fibrosis (MDE) [117].

Heart Failure with preserved Ejection Fraction

HFpEH accounts for half of all cases with heart failure [118]. It is characterized by symptoms of heart failure with normal or mildly reduced LVEF and evidence of diastolic dysfunction [119]. Echocardiography has been the corner stone in the assessment of HFpEF, but CMR has an increasing and evolving role in the evaluation of these patients. CMR provides a highly reproducible method of assessment of the LV volume and LVEF, and therefore decreases the chance of misclassification of heart failure. CMR can also provide an accurate method for quantification of LV mass of and assessment of the extent and spatial distribution of LV hypertrophy. LV mass assessment by CMR has been validated in autopsy specimens [120] and is currently the gold standard in measuring LV and RV mass [121]. Conversely, the role of CMR in evaluation of diastolic function is limited. Although peak early and late LV filling rate and time to peak of LV filling can be measured owing the high spatial resolution of CMR, the utility of these measures is limited due to time consuming analysis [122]. Similarly, the use of CMR tagging to evaluate ventricular untwisting is far from clinical implementation. The utilization of the other measures of diastolic function such as CMR Velocity-encoded imaging or tissue-phase mapping is limited by the lower temporal resolution compared to echocardiography [123].

Hypertrophic Cardiomyopathy

Hypertrophic cardiomyopathy (HCM) is a genetic cardiomyopathy with variable phenotypic expression. The most common phenotype is asymmetrical LV hypertrophy, but it can present as a symmetrical form, apical form or in an end-stage form with LV thinning and systolic dysfunction (burned-out HCM) [124]. CMR performs better than echocardiography in diagnosing HCM and in evaluation of the location and extent of the hypertrophy particularly, the apical form [125 - 128]. Equivalently, CMR better detects associated apical aneurysms associated with adverse events [129]. It can accurately measure the exact septal thickness, systolic anterior mitral leaflet motion and detect papillary muscles that are associated with left ventricular outflow tract (LVOT) obstruction [130, 131].

The pattern of MDE in HCM is diverse in location and pattern but most frequently seen as patchy midwall at the RV insertion point. Although it is mostly seen in areas with hypertrophy but it has been observed in segments with normal wall thickness (Fig. **4**) [126, 132]. MDE is an independent predictor of sudden cardiac death even in the absence of other conventional markers [133]. The presence of MDE is associated with a higher risk of ventricular arrhythmia on 24-hour Holter and the absence of MDE incurs a very low risk of events [133]. Furthermore, MDE was associated with a 7-fold increase in the risk of nonsustained ventricular tachycardia [134].

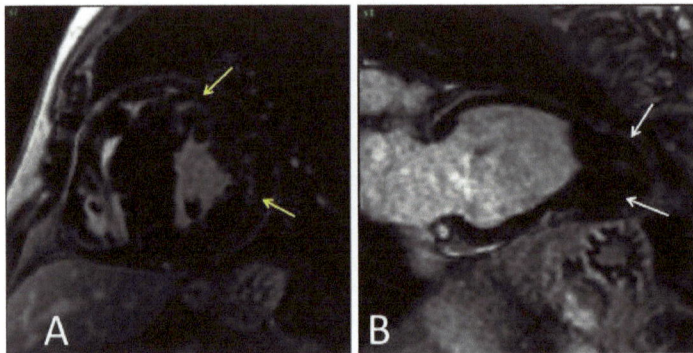

Fig. (4). Delayed myocardial enhancement images showing typical appearance of hypertrophic cardiomyopathy with midwall patch delayed enhancement in the right ventricle insertion point (*yellow arrows in figure A*) and the apical form of hypertrophic cardiomyopathy (*white arrows in figure B*).

Anderson-Fabry Disease

Anderson-Fabry disease (AFD) is an X-linked glycolipid storage disease due to abnormal lysosomal metabolism and characterized by accumulation of glycosphingolipid within the blood vessels and heart with subsequent LV hypertrophy (LVH) [135]. The disease should be suspected in any case of unexplained LVH particularly in young subjects as it is commonly mistaken as HCM [136]. Distinction between the two cases is of paramount clinical significance since AFD is a treatable condition and responds well to enzyme replacement therapy [137]. MDE is frequent finding in AFD [138, 139] and characteristically involves the epicardium of the basal and mid segments of the anterolateral and inferolateral walls [140].

Cardiac Amyloidosis

Cardiac involvement with amyloidosis is very common in AL amyloidosis (50%)

and frequently present as heart failure [141]. The prognosis of cardiac amyloidosis is generally poor and therefore prompt diagnosis is crucial to improve survival [142]. Although amyloidosis is a systemic disease, cardiac involvement can be the first manifestation of the disease [143]. CMR has emerged as new non-invasive tool for the diagnosis of cardiac amyloidosis. It can show the classical findings of LVH, thick atrial septum, bi-atrial dilatation as well as the presence of pericardial effusion, MDE has variable appearance in amyloidosis, it can be seen as a circumferential subendocardial enhancement of the LV, a zebra-stripe appearance with subendocardial enhancement of the LV and RV or patchy transmural appearance. In some cases, it is difficult to determine the right inversion time for the MDE due to rapid exchange of gadolinium between blood pool and amyloid fibrils within the myocardium [141, 144, 145]. In one study, the subendocardial MDE has a sensitivity of 80% and specificity 94% of in diagnosing amyloidosis [143]. The presence MDE correlates well with heart failure severity (B-type natriuretic peptide) and survival in patients with cardiac amyloidosis [146, 147].

Arrhythmogenic Right Ventricular Cardiomyopathy

Arrhythmogenic Right Ventricular Cardiomyopathy or Dysplasia (ARVC) maybe asymptomatic or may present with heart failure, sudden cardiac death or ventricular arrhythmia [148]. It is characterized by fibrofatty replacement of the RV myocardium but can affect both ventricles [149 - 151]. CMR is an integral part of the proposed modified task force criteria for the diagnosis of ARVC. These include RV wall motion abnormalities with RV dilatation. Regional RV akinesia or dyskinesia or dyssynchronous RV contraction, and one of the following ratio of RV end-diastolic volume to BSA 110 mL/m2 (male) or 100 mL/m^2 (female), or RV ejection fraction 40% constitutes a major criterion, while regional RV akinesia or dyskinesia or dyssynchronous RV contraction and one of the following: whether ratio of RV end-diastolic volume to BSA 100 to 110 mL/m^2 (male) or 90 to 100 mL/m^2 (female) or RV ejection fraction > 40% to ≤ 45% constitutes a minor criterion [152]. Although the presence of MDE is neither a major or a minor criterion for the diagnosis of ARVC due to its low sensitivity, specificity and reproducibility [153], MDE itself correlates well with fibrofatty replacement on endomyocardial biopsy and predicts inducible ventricular tachycardia during electrophysiological studies [154].

Constrictive Pericarditis

Constrictive pericarditis presents with symptoms of heart failure despite normal LVEF. CMR provides accurate morphological assessment of the pericardium such as pericardial thickening . Pericardial thickness >4mm is highly suggestive of constriction an can help differentiating constrictive pericarditis from constrictive cardiomyopathy by CMR (93% diagnostic accuracy) [155]. Cine images may also show the characteristic morphological appearance of the atria and ventricles; dilated atria and elongated tubular ventricles [156]. Tissue characterization with edema and delayed enhancement images provide information about the presence and extent of inflammation and fibrosis and whether it is acute or chronic. Real-time cine images can demonstrate inter-ventricular dependence [157]. CMR is also used to monitor response to therapy in some case with transient constrictive pericarditis.

CMR in the Advanced Care of Heart Failure

As discussed earlier, CMR plays a crucial role in clinical decision-making regarding AICD implantation by accurate evaluation of LVEF. Some studies have further suggested that CMR may play a role in the selection of patients for cardiac resynchronization therapy (CRT). ICM, number of viable segments, large scar burden and scar location such as septum or posterolateral wall are associated with limited response to CRT [158 - 161]. CMR also has a promising potential in follow up of patients post cardiac transplant; CAD associated with cardiac transplant can be detected by MDE and there are early reports to suggest detection of rejection by T2-weighted images [162]. Finally, stem cell therapy is a promising treatment option for patients with advanced heart failure. Owing its high spatial resolution and ability to detect small changes in EF, CMR may be used in follow up of patient with cell therapy [20, 163].

Future Application of CMR

Despite the well-established application of CMR in heart failure, its role is continuously evolving. The main future development is CMR is the move towards quantification rather than visual assessment of regional MDE. T1 mapping is a technique that allows CMR to evaluate diffuse subclinical fibrosis in the myocardium, which can be obtained with or with GBCA [164, 165]. It allows an accurate quantification of extracellular volume [166] which is shown to add diagnostic and prognostic value in heart failure with reduced and preserved ejection fraction [167, 168]. Time resolved, 3D phase contrast flow (4D flow) imaging is another novel technique that allows visualization of velocity and direction of blood flow and quantization of hemodynamic parameters such as wall shear stress and may play a an important role in CMR evaluation of aortopathy and congenital heart disease [169, 170]. Finally, diffusion tensor imaging allows for non-invasive assessment the microstructure of the myocardium and appears to be promising in the evaluation of remodeling after myocardial infarction [171].

CARDIAC COMPUTED TOMOGRAPHY

The introduction of 64-row Multidetector Computed Tomography (MDCT) has significantly increased the utility of cardiac computed tomography (CCT) in contemporary cardiac practice. Cardiac computed tomography angiography (CCTA) has emerged as a valuable non-invasive diagnostic and prognostic tool in evaluation of CAD [172, 173]. However, CCT has an evolving role in management of patient of heart failure.

CCT Techniques and Protocols

CCT is a non-invasive test that utilizes ionizing radiation to image the heart from different angles simultaneously. These images are computer processed resulting in 3D image of the cardiac structures. ECG gating is used to determine the time of systole and diastole as well as the best time for imaging the coronary arteries. ECG gating can be either prospective or retrospective with differences in radiation exposure [174, 175] In order to decrease the motion artifact, the patients are asked to hold their breath to eliminate respiratory motion; in addition, beta-blockers are used to decrease the heart rate in order to minimize cardiac motion. Additionally, sublingual nitroglycerin is given to dilate the coronary arteries prior to image acquisition.

The imaging protocol includes quantification of coronary artery calcification (CAC) [176], coronary artery angiography and evaluation of other cardiac structure as well as the major vessels. CAC quantification is performed without contrast administration. Coronary angiography is performed with iodinated contrast agent. Serum creatinine and glomerular filtration rate (GFR) should be checked before administrating of the contrast agent. Contrast induced nephropathy (CIN) remains a risk even in patients with normal renal function since advanced heart failure is considered a risk factor for CIN [177]. Since CCT utilizes ionized radiation, it is relatively contraindicated during pregnancy. However, recent advances in hardware and imaging protocols have significantly lowered the radiation dose [178, 179].

Coronary Artery Calcification and Evaluation of Heart Failure

CAC is a measure of subclinical atherosclerosis. The presence of a non-zero CAC score has been associated with a high likelihood of significant CAD and the absence of CAC is associated with a very low probability of significant CAD [180 - 182]. Therefore, CAC can be used to differentiate ischemic and non-ischemic cardiomyopathy. In a study of 120 patients with heart failure, CAC was associated with a high sensitivity (>90%) in detection of ICM [183]. Moreover, CAC performs better than echocardiography in detection of ICM [184]. But more importantly, a CAC> 400 is associated with a hazard ratio of 4 in predicting heart failure [185].

Cardiac Computed Tomography Angiography and Etiology of Heart Failure

Cardiac Computed Tomography Angiography (CCTA) is increasingly used to differentiate ischemic from non-ischemic cardiomyopathy especially in patients with low likelihood of having CAD. CCTA is a robust non-invasive modality for the diagnosis of CAD owing its high specificity and negative predictive value (NPV). Multiple studies have demonstrated the diagnostic accuracy of CCTA (sensitivity of 95-99%), particularly the high NPV (97-99%) in ruling out CAD and therefore it as an excellent choice as a rule-out modality [172, 186]. The diagnostic accuracy of CCTA to rule-out CAD in patients with newly diagnosed DCM was 94% in comparison to ICA (Fig. **5**) [187, 188]. Recent advances in the CT evaluation of fluid dynamics allowed for the introduction of CT functional flow reserve that added a functional assessment to the evaluation of anatomic stenosis, further improving the diagnostic accuracy of CCTA [189, 190]. The initial experience of CT myocardial perfusion in detection of CAD is encouraging [191]. However, the role of the two latter techniques in heart failure has not been evaluated yet. Given all of the above, the Appropriateness Use Criteria (AUC) considers the use of CCTA in the initial evaluation of ischemic etiology of heart failure as appropriate [192].

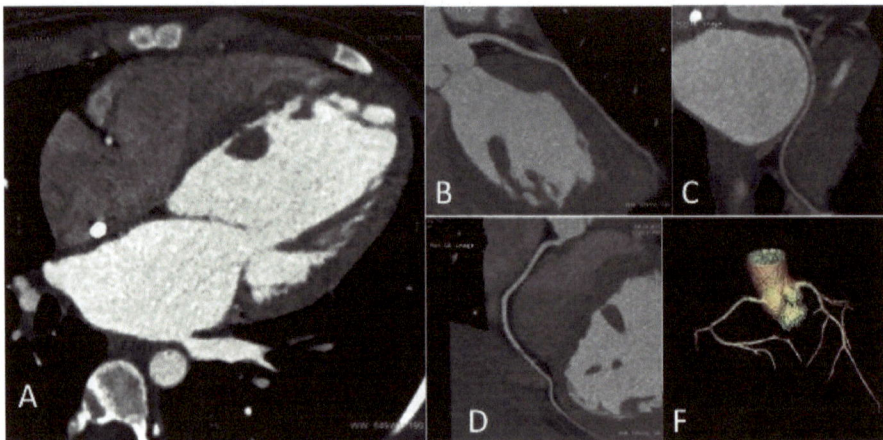

Fig. (5). Cardiac CTA of a patient with new onset heart failure showing dilated LV (A), and normal coronary arteries (LAD (B), (LCx) C, RCA (D) and F).

Furthermore, CCTA has a potential role in the evaluation of LVNC. Similar to CMR, an end-diastolic noncompacted/compacted ratio of more than 2.3 was suggested to diagnose LVNC on CCTA [193].

CCT also provides accurate morphological assessment of the pericardium in cases of constrictive pericarditis [156]. CCT has higher sensitivity for the detection and evaluation of pericardial calcification. Pericardial calcification is associated with the diagnosis of constrictive pericarditis, but absence of calcification does not exclude the diagnosis [155]. CCT also provides valuable information about for preoperative planning by localization and extent of pericardial calcification.

Cardiac Computed Tomography Angiography and Assessment of LV Volume and Ejection Fraction

The CCT has the highest spatial resolution among the various cardiac imaging modalities which gives the advantage of accurate assessment of the LV wall thickness and size and allows an accurate evaluation of CAD complication such as wall thinning and development of LV aneurysm and pseudoaneurysm [194, 195]. Multiple studies have demonstrated the accuracy of CCT in the evaluation of LV volumes and ejection fraction. There was a good correlation found between CCT and CMR in evaluation of both LVEF (r =0.97) and RVEF (r =0.86) [196]. CCT showed lower LVEF and higher LV volumes in comparison to other modalities [197], Moreover, the relation between CCT and echocardiography measurements was better in dilated LV compared to non-dilated LV [198]. However, these studies were performed with retrospective ECG gating which is associated with high radiation dose. Nonetheless, a recent study has demonstrated the feasibility and accuracy of low radiation dose CCT in the evaluation of LVEF in comparison to nuclear radionuclide angiography [199]. CCT has also been useful in detection of cardiac thrombi. The high spatial resolution allows for the diagnosis of layered clots that take the shape of the inner contour of the LV making it difficult to detect by echocardiography. The thrombi typically have lower attenuation than the myocardium [200]. Moreover, CCT has been shown to be of value in ruling out thrombi in the left atrium (LA) and left atrial appendage (LAA) prior to atrial fibrillation ablation [201, 202].

CCT and Evaluation of Infarct Size and Myocardial Scar

CCT can be used in the evaluation of myocardial scar and assessment of viability. Delayed myocardial enhancement by CCT (MDE-CT) has been recently used in evaluation of myocardial scar. In chronic myocardial infarction, the iodinated contrast accumulates in the myocardial interstitium similar to delayed myocardial enhancement by CMR (MDE CMR). Myocardial scar has higher attenuation (higher Hounsfield Unit (HU)) than normal myocardium in images obtained 5-10 minutes after administration of the contract. Excellent correlation was demonstrated between MDE-CT and histopathology in animal model [203]. Similar agreement was demonstrated between MDE-CT and MDE-CMR in evaluation of chronic MI in humans [204, 205]. However, the superior spatial resolution of MDCT allows for better delineation of the extent of the infarct. Good agreement was also demonstrated between MDE-CT and dobutamine stress echocardiography [206]. New Hardware technologies allow for color coded map of iodine density through the use of dual-source scanners and therefore gives a better assessment of the extent of the infarct [207]. The role of CCT in evaluation of myocardial scar and viability is evolving and awaits more studies before routine implementation of this technology in clinical practice.

CCT and the Advanced Care of Heart Failure

Although CCTA has limited role in the decision of device therapy in heart failure, it can be used in mapping of the cardiac venous system to help in the implantation of the LV lead in cardiac resynchronization therapy (CRT) [208]. In CRT, pacing the LV is achieved via a lead that goes through one of the cardiac veins which has considerable variation in number and course [209]. Atrial fibrillation (AF) is very common in heart failure [210]. LAA occluder devices were recently approved for prevention of the thromboembolism in patients with AF [211]. CCT can provide accurate 3D evaluation of the size of the body and neck of the LAA, which are crucial for successful exclusion and anchoring of the device [212, 213]. Recently, CCTA has been used for non-invasive evaluation of left ventricular assessed devices (LVAD). CCTA can provide information about the position of the outflow cannula causes of low LVAD reading, diagnosis of LVAD thrombosis and pre-surgical planning [214, 215].

Future Application of CCTA

With the advances in technology, cardiac CT will be possibly done by ultralow radiation dose and contrast volume [216 - 218]. Preliminary work on CCT and regenerative cell therapy showed promising results as CCT was useful in evaluating infarct size and LVEF following stem cell transplant [219]. In addition, there is a lot of ongoing research in hybrid imaging (CCTA and nuclear imaging), CCT myocardial perfusion and tissue characterization, which has promising potential in evaluation and prognostication of patient with heart failure.

NUCLEAR SCINTIGRAPHY

The contemporary understanding of heart failure describes a combination of molecular, neurohormonal and structural changes that ends in the clinical syndrome of pump failure and fluid imbalance that can be cause numerous etiologies. Among the various imaging modalities, nuclear cardiology has the highest sensitivity in evaluation of molecular changes in addition to investigating causes, status and prognosis of heart failure [220 - 222].

Nuclear Cardiology Techniques and Protocols

Various protocols and radioactive tracers are employed in nuclear cardiology. Two main technologies are used; Single Photon Emission Tomography (SPECT) which uses gamma camera to detect gamma rays emitted from a radioactive isotope that bound to the heart after being injected into the patient allowing for functional imaging [223], and Positron Emission Tomography (PET) which utilizes special radiotracers that emits positrons and allows for functional and metabolic imaging. Various protocols are used depending of on the clinical indication. In ischemia evaluation, vasodilator or dobutamine are used to stress the patient and demonstrate ischemia. Radiotracer is injected at rest and peak heart rate (in case of dobutamine) or pea hyperemia (in case of vasodilator), ischemia is then detected by comparing stress and rest images [224]. Addition of ECG-gating provide additional information about wall motion and LVEF [225]. In addition to ischemia evaluation, metabolic imaging with 18-flurodeoxyglocose permits differentiation between infracted and hibernating myocardium by PET [226]. These tests are associated with exposure to ionizing radiation that is more significant in SPECT compared to PET. However, new advancements in SPECT have significant impact in radiation dose reduction [227, 228].

Nuclear Cardiology and evaluation of Left ventricular Ejection Fraction

Radionuclide Angiography and Left Ventricular Function

Radionuclide angiography (RNA) has been used for assessment of LV for decades [229]. During the test right blood cells (RBC) are labeled with radioactive tracer and the ECG-gated images are obtained throughout the cardiac cycle. The LVEF and RVEF are measured at the equilibrium state by tracing the cavity in end-systole and end-diastole and the EF is calculated form the difference radioactivity between the two readings. Therefore, RNA allows for evaluation of LV volume and LVEF independent of geometric assumption resulting in a highly accurate measurement. Hence, RNA is used in clinical decision making in cases of chemotherapy induced LV dysfunction and timing of AICD implantation [230, 231]. First pass RNA measures the nuclear activity of the RV and LV in the first few beats, thereby allowing measurement of systolic function of both ventricle as well as valvular regurgitation. Moreover, LV dyssynchrony and diastolic dysfunction can be evaluated by measurement of cyclic radioactivity variation [232].

SPECT and PET and Left Ventricular Function

Using ECG-gating during SPECT and PET image acquisition permits identification of systole and diastole during cardiac cycle. Automatic algorithms are then employed to detect wall motion and quantify LVEF at rest and post stress [233, 234]. The accuracy of SPECT derived LVEF has been demonstrated against RNA and CMR. There was an excellent correlation between SPECT and RNA derived LVEF (r=0.93) [235]. Similarly, there was a close correlation (r= 0.75-0.85) between SPECT and CMR derived LVEF [236]. Equivalently, PET has reasonable correlation to CMR derived LVEF (r=0.63-0.99) [237]. Quantification of LVEF Both SPECT and PET provide additional prognostic information, post-stress EF has been shown to be a strong predictor of cardiac death [238].

Nuclear Cardiology and Etiology of Heart Failure

Nuclear Myocardial Perfusion Imaging (MPI) is the most widely used non-invasive test for the diagnosis of CAD. Its use is supported with a wealth of evidence proving its diagnostic and prognostic value.

Pooled data from various SPECT stress protocols revealed a sensitivity of 90% and specificity of around 80% in detection of significant CAD [239], making it an accurate test for the evaluation of patients with new onset heart failure and low likelihood of CAD. Furthermore, significant perfusion defects on SPECT were associated with the new onset and refractory heart failure in general population [240] as well as with mortality in patients with ischemic CMP [241].

Similarly, cardiac PET has high diagnostic accuracy in the diagnosis of CAD. PET performs better than SPECT with a sensitivity and specificity of 90% and 88% respectively [242]. Additionally, PET allows for measurement of myocardial blood flow and flow reserve, which is a marker of poor prognosis in patients with ischemic and idiopathic CMP [243, 244]. Impaired myocardial blood flow was a stronger predictor of cardiac death compared to LVEF (HR of 4.11 *Vs* 2.76) [245]. Moreover, reduced myocardial flow reserve was also shown to be a predictor of ventricular arrhythmia, cardiac death, heart failure hospitalization, late revascularization, and aborted sudden cardiac death [244, 246].

Nuclear Cardiology and Evaluation of Myocardial Scar and Viability

Assessment of myocardial viability is of paramount importance in clinical decision making related to revascularization in patients with heart failure and CAD. While revascularization in patients with evidence of viability is associated with significant reduction in cardiac death [247], revascularization of non-viable myocardium subject the patients for the risks associated with the procedure with no substantial benefits.

On SPECT, viability can be assessed with either [201]Thallium (^{201}Tl) or [99]Tichnecium (^{99}Tc) based tracers. Viability assessment by ^{201}Tl depends on two characteristics of ^{201}Tl uptake; the uptake of ^{201}Tl is an energy-dependent process requiring intact cell membrane and the redistribution properties of ^{201}Tl, in which there is a late distribution of tracer to areas of viable myocardium that has no uptake in the early stage [248]. The protocol involves early and late (24hour) imaging of the myocardium, so segments that have early tracer uptake and segments that have uptake in the late redistribution images are viable. Unlike ^{201}Tl, ^{99}Tc does not exhibit redistribution property; so segments that have tracer uptake are viable. SPECT has 70-80% sensitivity in detecting myocardial viability [249]. However, low spatial resolution and attenuation artifacts limit the diagnostic accuracy [250]. Around 45% of the segments deemed non-viable by ^{201}TI have demonstrated evidence uptake after revascularization [251].

Evaluation of viability by PET is performed through metabolic imaging with 18-flurodeoxyglocose (^{18}FDG) in comparison to reset perfusion images. Normally myocardial cells utilize fatty acid to produce energy; however, chronically ischemic cells shift to glucose metabolism. Hence, there is uptake of ^{18}FDG despite the absence of uptake in rest perfusion images. The areas that show mismatched uptake are considered viable while areas that have matched defects are considered as non-viable (Figs. **6** and **7**). Cardiac PET has high diagnostic accuracy in predicting recovery after revascularization (85-90% sensitivity) [252]. The degree of improvement of LVEF is related to the extent of mismatch on PET [253]. Moreover, measurement of myocardial blood flow may have value in predicting LV recovery [249]. However, glucose resistance and abnormal glucose metabolism in diabetic patients may limit the diagnostic accuracy of ^{18}FDG PET.

Nuclear Cardiology and Sarcoidosis

^{18}FDG PET can be used to detect areas of active inflammation within myocardium [254]. Cells with active inflammation utilize glucose to meet their high metabolic demands. Therefore, combination of the ^{18}FDG and rest perfusion PET images provides a tool for the diagnosis, prognosis in cardiac sarcoidosis. Pooled data revealed a sensitivity of 89% and specificity of 78% of ^{18}FDG PET in diagnosis of cardiac sarcoidosis [255]. Although both CMR and ^{18}FDG PET can be used in the diagnosis cardiac sarcoidosis, ^{18}FDG PET has the advantage of being performed in patients with cardiac devices. Active inflammation detected with ^{18}FDG PET is associated with higher risk of ventricular arrhythmia requiring AICD shock in patients with sarcoidosis [256] and can be used to monitor response to steroid therapy [257].

Imaging of Cardiac Innervations

The neurohormonal imbalance in heart failure results in downregulation of B-adrenergic receptors resulting in catecholamine toxicity that further worsens LV function [258]. Hence, evaluation of the sympathetic innervation may predict response to B- blocker therapy [259]. Moreover, Increased cardiac sympathetic innervation and autonomic dysfunction has been linked to mortality in patients with heart failure irrespective of etiology [260]. ^{123}I-metaiodobenzylguanidine (^{123}I-MIBG) imaging by SPECT has enabled direct evaluation of overall cardiac sympathetic function. ^{123}I-MIBG is an analogue of the false neurotransmitter, guanetidine, a potent selective sympathetic neuron-blocking agent. Cardiac evaluation by ^{123}I-MIBG includes cardiac retention by calculating heart mediastinal ratio (HMR) and cardiac washout [261]. Both parameters have been shown to predict worsening HF, life-threatening arrhythmias, and sudden cardiac death in chronic HF [262]. ^{11}C-hydroxyephedrine (^{11}C-HED) is used to image the sympathetic innervation of the heart. The uptake of ^{11}C-HED has been shown to be reduced in LV dysfunction [222].

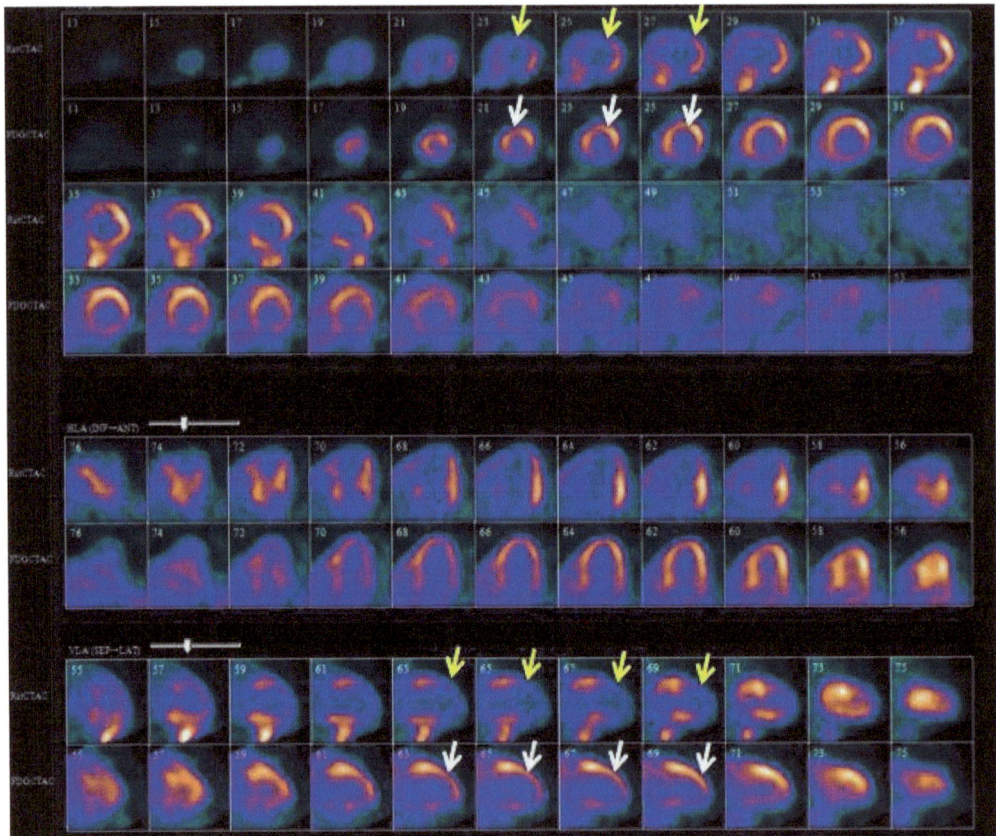

Fig. (6). [18]FDG PET viability study showing matched perfusion (severe perfusion defect in rest Rubidium perfusion images (*yellow arrows*) and [18]FDG perfusion (*white arrows*) indicating non-viable LAD territory.

Nuclear Cardiology and Molecular Imaging

Multiple radiotracers are currently being investigated for molecular imaging of various pathologies entities in heart failure. These tracers provide valuable insights of the presence and magnitude of different pathological processes including cell necrosis [263], cellular apoptosis which has a special application in detection of rejection post cardiac transplant [264], and extracellular fibrosis, fibrogenesis and matrix degeneration. However, most of these tracers are not available for clinical use [220].

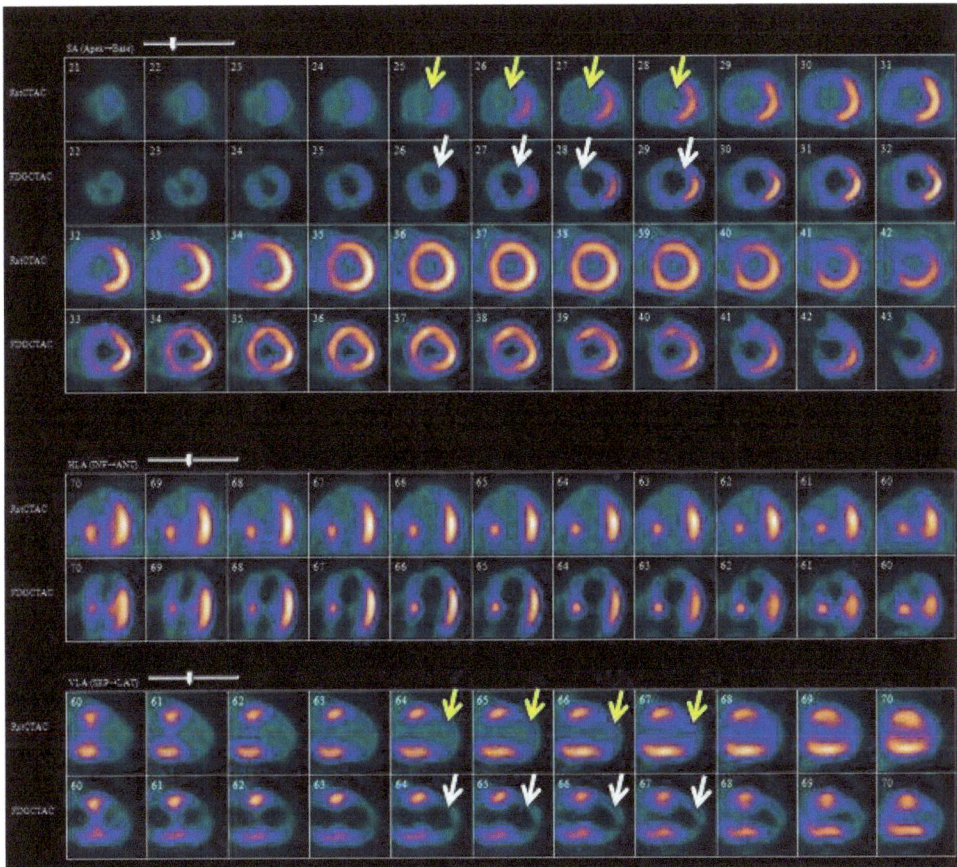

Fig. (7). ^{18}FDG PET viability study showing mismatched perfusion (severe perfusion defect in rest Rubidium perfusion images (*yellow arrows*) and normal^{18}FDG perfusion (*white arrows*) indicating hibernation of the LAD territory.

Future Application of Nuclear Cardiology

Current research in nuclear cardiology concentrates in reduction of radiation dose, improving the diagnostic accuracy of SPECT with the addition CT attenuation correction and development of new tracers. In heart failure, there is ongoing work with molecular imaging for better visualization of pathophysiological processes. Finally, there are major developments in hybrid imaging combining the anatomical imaging by CCTA with the functional imaging of nuclear cardiology.

CONCLUSION

Non-invasive cardiac imaging plays a pivotal role in the contemporary care of heart failure. It has a tremendous potential for better comprehension of the mechanism of heart failure, detection of subclinical disease, assessment and classification of the current state of the established disease and provision of insights regarding prognosis and response to therapy. CMR, CCT and nuclear cardiology provide robust diagnostic and prognostic information offering the physician with a detailed insight in many aspects of the heart failure management. CMR provides the most comprehensive information but it is limited by the availability. Nuclear cardiology particularly PET provides high diagnostic yield and has exceptional potential particularly in molecular imaging, but is limited by the ionizing radiation and limited availability of PET. CCTA has an established role in diagnosis of CAD and evolving role in tissue characterization, but like nuclear cardiology limited by associated radiation. Recent advances and ongoing research is expanding the utility of cardiac imaging and its use is likely to increase with the epidemic of heart failure.

CONSENT FOR PUBLICATION

Not applicable.

CONFLICT OF INTEREST

The authors confirm that this chapter contents have no conflict of interest.

ACKNOWLEDGEMENTS

Declared none.

REFERENCES

[1]   Yancy CW, Jessup M, Bozkurt B, *et al.* 2013 ACCF/AHA guideline for the management of heart failure: a report of the American College of Cardiology Foundation/American Heart Association Task Force on practice guidelines. Circulation 2013; 128(16): e240-327.
[http://dx.doi.org/10.1161/CIR.0b013e31829e8776] [PMID: 23741058]

[2]   McMurray JJ, Adamopoulos S, Anker SD, *et al.* ESC Guidelines for the diagnosis and treatment of acute and chronic heart failure 2012: The Task Force for the Diagnosis and Treatment of Acute and Chronic Heart Failure 2012 of the European Society of Cardiology. Developed in collaboration with the Heart Failure Association (HFA) of the ESC. Eur Heart J 2012; 33(14): 1787-847.

[http://dx.doi.org/10.1093/eurheartj/ehs104] [PMID: 22611136]

[3]   Go AS, Mozaffarian D, Roger VL, *et al.* Heart disease and stroke statistics--2013 update: a report from the American Heart Association. Circulation 2013; 127(1): e6-e245.
[http://dx.doi.org/10.1161/CIR.0b013e31828124ad] [PMID: 23239837]

[4]   Roger VL, Weston SA, Redfield MM, *et al.* Trends in heart failure incidence and survival in a community-based population. JAMA 2004; 292(3): 344-50.
[http://dx.doi.org/10.1001/jama.292.3.344] [PMID: 15265849]

[5]   Hendel RC, Patel MR, Kramer CM, *et al.* ACCF/ACR/SCCT/SCMR/ASNC/NASCI/SCAI/SIR 2006 appropriateness criteria for cardiac computed tomography and cardiac magnetic resonance imaging: a report of the American College of Cardiology Foundation Quality Strategic Directions Committee Appropriateness Criteria Working Group, American College of Radiology, Society of Cardiovascular Computed Tomography, Society for Cardiovascular Magnetic Resonance, American Society of Nuclear Cardiology, North American Society for Cardiac Imaging, Society for Cardiovascular Angiography and Interventions, and Society of Interventional Radiology. J Am Coll Cardiol 2006; 48(7): 1475-97.
[http://dx.doi.org/10.1016/j.jacc.2006.07.003] [PMID: 17010819]

[6]   Pennell DJ, Sechtem UP, Higgins CB, *et al.* Clinical indications for cardiovascular magnetic resonance (CMR): Consensus Panel report. Eur Heart J 2004; 25(21): 1940-65.
[http://dx.doi.org/10.1016/j.ehj.2004.06.040] [PMID: 15522474]

[7]   Kramer CM, Barkhausen J, Flamm SD, Kim RJ, Nagel E. Standardized cardiovascular magnetic resonance (CMR) protocols 2013 update. J Cardiovasc Magn Reson 2013; 15: 91.
[http://dx.doi.org/10.1186/1532-429X-15-91] [PMID: 24103764]

[8]   Doltra A, Amundsen BH, Gebker R, Fleck E, Kelle S. Emerging concepts for myocardial late gadolinium enhancement MRI. Curr Cardiol Rev 2013; 9(3): 185-90.
[http://dx.doi.org/10.2174/1573403X113099990030] [PMID: 23909638]

[9]   Sakuma H. Coronary CT *versus* MR angiography: the role of MR angiography. Radiology 2011; 258(2): 340-9.
[http://dx.doi.org/10.1148/radiol.10100116] [PMID: 21273518]

[10]   Mostbeck GH, Caputo GR, Higgins CB. MR measurement of blood flow in the cardiovascular system. AJR Am J Roentgenol 1992; 159(3): 453-61.
[http://dx.doi.org/10.2214/ajr.159.3.1503004] [PMID: 1503004]

[11]   Cawley PJ, Maki JH, Otto CM. Cardiovascular magnetic resonance imaging for valvular heart disease: technique and validation. Circulation 2009; 119(3): 468-78.
[http://dx.doi.org/10.1161/CIRCULATIONAHA.107.742486] [PMID: 19171869]

[12]   Kuo PH, Kanal E, Abu-Alfa AK, Cowper SE. Gadolinium-based MR contrast agents and nephrogenic systemic fibrosis. Radiology 2007; 242(3): 647-9.
[http://dx.doi.org/10.1148/radiol.2423061640] [PMID: 17213364]

[13]   Shellock FG, Crues JV. MR procedures: biologic effects, safety, and patient care. Radiology 2004; 232(3): 635-52.
[http://dx.doi.org/10.1148/radiol.2323030830] [PMID: 15284433]

[14]   Moss AJ, Kutyifa V. Safe MRI in Patients With an Upgraded (Conditional) Implantable Cardioverter-Defibrillator: The Beneficial Tip of a Troublesome Iceberg. J Am Coll Cardiol 2015; 65(24): 2589-90.
[http://dx.doi.org/10.1016/j.jacc.2015.04.048] [PMID: 25982015]

[15]   Curtis JP, Sokol SI, Wang Y, *et al.* The association of left ventricular ejection fraction, mortality, and cause of death in stable outpatients with heart failure. J Am Coll Cardiol 2003; 42(4): 736-42.
[http://dx.doi.org/10.1016/S0735-1097(03)00789-7] [PMID: 12932612]

[16]   Epstein AE, DiMarco JP, Ellenbogen KA, *et al.* 2012 ACCF/AHA/HRS focused update incorporated into the ACCF/AHA/HRS 2008 guidelines for device-based therapy of cardiac rhythm abnormalities:

a report of the American College of Cardiology Foundation/American Heart Association Task Force on Practice Guidelines and the Heart Rhythm Society. J Am Coll Cardiol 2013; 61(3): e6-e75.
[http://dx.doi.org/10.1016/j.jacc.2012.11.007] [PMID: 23265327]

[17]   Dickstein K, Vardas PE, Auricchio A, *et al.* 2010 Focused Update of ESC Guidelines on device therapy in heart failure: an update of the 2008 ESC Guidelines for the diagnosis and treatment of acute and chronic heart failure and the 2007 ESC guidelines for cardiac and resynchronization therapy. Developed with the special contribution of the Heart Failure Association and the European Heart Rhythm Association. Eur Heart J 2010; 31(21): 2677-87.
[http://dx.doi.org/10.1093/eurheartj/ehq337] [PMID: 20801924]

[18]   Bernard Y, Meneveau N, Boucher S, *et al.* Lack of agreement between left ventricular volumes and ejection fraction determined by two-dimensional echocardiography and contrast cineangiography in postinfarction patients. Echocardiography 2001; 18(2): 113-22.
[http://dx.doi.org/10.1046/j.1540-8175.2001.00113.x] [PMID: 11262534]

[19]   Bellenger NG, Burgess MI, Ray SG, *et al.* Comparison of left ventricular ejection fraction and volumes in heart failure by echocardiography, radionuclide ventriculography and cardiovascular magnetic resonance; are they interchangeable? Eur Heart J 2000; 21(16): 1387-96.
[http://dx.doi.org/10.1053/euhj.2000.2011] [PMID: 10952828]

[20]   Karamitsos TD, Francis JM, Myerson S, Selvanayagam JB, Neubauer S. The role of cardiovascular magnetic resonance imaging in heart failure. J Am Coll Cardiol 2009; 54(15): 1407-24.
[http://dx.doi.org/10.1016/j.jacc.2009.04.094] [PMID: 19796734]

[21]   Walsh TF, Hundley WG. Assessment of ventricular function with cardiovascular magnetic resonance. Cardiol Clin 2007; 25(1): 15-33, v. [v.].
[http://dx.doi.org/10.1016/j.ccl.2007.01.002] [PMID: 17478238]

[22]   Selvanayagam J, Westaby S, Channon K, *et al.* Images in cardiovascular medicine. Surgical left ventricular restoration: an extreme case. Circulation 2003; 107(10)e71
[http://dx.doi.org/10.1161/01.CIR.0000056080.19298.56] [PMID: 12642370]

[23]   Karamitsos TD, Hudsmith LE, Selvanayagam JB, Neubauer S, Francis JM. Operator induced variability in left ventricular measurements with cardiovascular magnetic resonance is improved after training. J Cardiovasc Magn Reson 2007; 9(5): 777-83.
[http://dx.doi.org/10.1080/10976640701545073] [PMID: 17891615]

[24]   Mahrholdt H, Wagner A, Holly TA, *et al.* Reproducibility of chronic infarct size measurement by contrast-enhanced magnetic resonance imaging. Circulation 2002; 106(18): 2322-7.
[http://dx.doi.org/10.1161/01.CIR.0000036368.63317.1C] [PMID: 12403661]

[25]   Sarwar A, Shapiro MD, Abbara S, Cury RC. Cardiac magnetic resonance imaging for the evaluation of ventricular function. Semin Roentgenol 2008; 43(3): 183-92.
[http://dx.doi.org/10.1053/j.ro.2008.02.004] [PMID: 18486680]

[26]   Strohm O, Schulz-Menger J, Pilz B, Osterziel KJ, Dietz R, Friedrich MG. Measurement of left ventricular dimensions and function in patients with dilated cardiomyopathy. J Magn Reson Imaging 2001; 13(3): 367-71.
[http://dx.doi.org/10.1002/jmri.1052] [PMID: 11241808]

[27]   Tracy CM, Epstein AE, Darbar D, *et al.* 2012 ACCF/AHA/HRS focused update of the 2008 guidelines for device-based therapy of cardiac rhythm abnormalities: a report of the American College of Cardiology Foundation/American Heart Association Task Force on Practice Guidelines and the Heart Rhythm Society. [corrected]. Circulation 2012; 126(14): 1784-800. [corrected].
[http://dx.doi.org/10.1161/CIR.0b013e3182618569] [PMID: 22965336]

[28]   Wong M, Staszewsky L, Latini R, *et al.* Severity of left ventricular remodeling defines outcomes and response to therapy in heart failure: Valsartan heart failure trial (Val-HeFT) echocardiographic data. J Am Coll Cardiol 2004; 43(11): 2022-7.
[http://dx.doi.org/10.1016/j.jacc.2003.12.053] [PMID: 15172407]

[29]   Sun JP, James KB, Yang XS, *et al.* Comparison of mortality rates and progression of left ventricular dysfunction in patients with idiopathic dilated cardiomyopathy and dilated *versus* nondilated right ventricular cavities. Am J Cardiol 1997; 80(12): 1583-7.
[http://dx.doi.org/10.1016/S0002-9149(97)00780-7] [PMID: 9416940]

[30]   de Groote P, Millaire A, Foucher-Hossein C, *et al.* Right ventricular ejection fraction is an independent predictor of survival in patients with moderate heart failure. J Am Coll Cardiol 1998; 32(4): 948-54.
[http://dx.doi.org/10.1016/S0735-1097(98)00337-4] [PMID: 9768716]

[31]   Ghio S, Gavazzi A, Campana C, *et al.* Independent and additive prognostic value of right ventricular systolic function and pulmonary artery pressure in patients with chronic heart failure. J Am Coll Cardiol 2001; 37(1): 183-8.
[http://dx.doi.org/10.1016/S0735-1097(00)01102-5] [PMID: 11153735]

[32]   Larose E, Ganz P, Reynolds HG, *et al.* Right ventricular dysfunction assessed by cardiovascular magnetic resonance imaging predicts poor prognosis late after myocardial infarction. J Am Coll Cardiol 2007; 49(8): 855-62.
[http://dx.doi.org/10.1016/j.jacc.2006.10.056] [PMID: 17320743]

[33]   Felker GM, Thompson RE, Hare JM, *et al.* Underlying causes and long-term survival in patients with initially unexplained cardiomyopathy. N Engl J Med 2000; 342(15): 1077-84.
[http://dx.doi.org/10.1056/NEJM200004133421502] [PMID: 10760308]

[34]   He J, Ogden LG, Bazzano LA, Vupputuri S, Loria C, Whelton PK. Risk factors for congestive heart failure in US men and women: NHANES I epidemiologic follow-up study. Arch Intern Med 2001; 161(7): 996-1002.
[http://dx.doi.org/10.1001/archinte.161.7.996] [PMID: 11295963]

[35]   Baldasseroni S, Opasich C, Gorini M, *et al.* Left bundle-branch block is associated with increased 1-year sudden and total mortality rate in 5517 outpatients with congestive heart failure: a report from the Italian network on congestive heart failure. Am Heart J 2002; 143(3): 398-405.
[http://dx.doi.org/10.1067/mhj.2002.121264] [PMID: 11868043]

[36]   Dries DL, Sweitzer NK, Drazner MH, Stevenson LW, Gersh BJ. Prognostic impact of diabetes mellitus in patients with heart failure according to the etiology of left ventricular systolic dysfunction. J Am Coll Cardiol 2001; 38(2): 421-8.
[http://dx.doi.org/10.1016/S0735-1097(01)01408-5] [PMID: 11499733]

[37]   Aaronson KD, Schwartz JS, Chen TM, Wong KL, Goin JE, Mancini DM. Development and prospective validation of a clinical index to predict survival in ambulatory patients referred for cardiac transplant evaluation. Circulation 1997; 95(12): 2660-7.
[http://dx.doi.org/10.1161/01.CIR.95.12.2660] [PMID: 9193435]

[38]   Rehwald WG, Fieno DS, Chen EL, Kim RJ, Judd RM. Myocardial magnetic resonance imaging contrast agent concentrations after reversible and irreversible ischemic injury. Circulation 2002; 105(2): 224-9.
[http://dx.doi.org/10.1161/hc0202.102016] [PMID: 11790705]

[39]   Wesbey GE, Higgins CB, McNamara MT, *et al.* Effect of gadolinium-DTPA on the magnetic relaxation times of normal and infarcted myocardium. Radiology 1984; 153(1): 165-9.
[http://dx.doi.org/10.1148/radiology.153.1.6473778] [PMID: 6473778]

[40]   Kim RJ, Chen EL, Lima JA, Judd RM. Myocardial Gd-DTPA kinetics determine MRI contrast enhancement and reflect the extent and severity of myocardial injury after acute reperfused infarction. Circulation 1996; 94(12): 3318-26.
[http://dx.doi.org/10.1161/01.CIR.94.12.3318] [PMID: 8989146]

[41]   McCrohon JA, Moon JC, Prasad SK, *et al.* Differentiation of heart failure related to dilated cardiomyopathy and coronary artery disease using gadolinium-enhanced cardiovascular magnetic resonance. Circulation 2003; 108(1): 54-9.

[http://dx.doi.org/10.1161/01.CIR.0000078641.19365.4C] [PMID: 12821550]

[42] Beltrami CA, Finato N, Rocco M, *et al.* Structural basis of end-stage failure in ischemic cardiomyopathy in humans. Circulation 1994; 89(1): 151-63.
[http://dx.doi.org/10.1161/01.CIR.89.1.151] [PMID: 8281642]

[43] Kim RJ, Fieno DS, Parrish TB, *et al.* Relationship of MRI delayed contrast enhancement to irreversible injury, infarct age, and contractile function. Circulation 1999; 100(19): 1992-2002.
[http://dx.doi.org/10.1161/01.CIR.100.19.1992] [PMID: 10556226]

[44] Mahrholdt H, Wagner A, Judd RM, Sechtem U, Kim RJ. Delayed enhancement cardiovascular magnetic resonance assessment of non-ischaemic cardiomyopathies. Eur Heart J 2005; 26(15): 1461-74.
[http://dx.doi.org/10.1093/eurheartj/ehi258] [PMID: 15831557]

[45] Wagner A, Mahrholdt H, Thomson L, *et al.* Effects of time, dose, and inversion time for acute myocardial infarct size measurements based on magnetic resonance imaging-delayed contrast enhancement. J Am Coll Cardiol 2006; 47(10): 2027-33.
[http://dx.doi.org/10.1016/j.jacc.2006.01.059] [PMID: 16697321]

[46] Kim RJ, Wu E, Rafael A, *et al.* The use of contrast-enhanced magnetic resonance imaging to identify reversible myocardial dysfunction. N Engl J Med 2000; 343(20): 1445-53.
[http://dx.doi.org/10.1056/NEJM200011163432003] [PMID: 11078769]

[47] Beek AM, Kühl HP, Bondarenko O, *et al.* Delayed contrast-enhanced magnetic resonance imaging for the prediction of regional functional improvement after acute myocardial infarction. J Am Coll Cardiol 2003; 42(5): 895-901.
[http://dx.doi.org/10.1016/S0735-1097(03)00835-0] [PMID: 12957439]

[48] Selvanayagam JB, Kardos A, Francis JM, *et al.* Value of delayed-enhancement cardiovascular magnetic resonance imaging in predicting myocardial viability after surgical revascularization. Circulation 2004; 110(12): 1535-41.
[http://dx.doi.org/10.1161/01.CIR.0000142045.22628.74] [PMID: 15353496]

[49] Aletras AH, Tilak GS, Natanzon A, *et al.* Retrospective determination of the area at risk for reperfused acute myocardial infarction with T2-weighted cardiac magnetic resonance imaging: histopathological and displacement encoding with stimulated echoes (DENSE) functional validations. Circulation 2006; 113(15): 1865-70.
[http://dx.doi.org/10.1161/CIRCULATIONAHA.105.576025] [PMID: 16606793]

[50] Friedrich MG, Abdel-Aty H, Taylor A, Schulz-Menger J, Messroghli D, Dietz R. The salvaged area at risk in reperfused acute myocardial infarction as visualized by cardiovascular magnetic resonance. J Am Coll Cardiol 2008; 51(16): 1581-7.
[http://dx.doi.org/10.1016/j.jacc.2008.01.019] [PMID: 18420102]

[51] Roes SD, Borleffs CJ, van der Geest RJ, *et al.* Infarct tissue heterogeneity assessed with contrast-enhanced MRI predicts spontaneous ventricular arrhythmia in patients with ischemic cardiomyopathy and implantable cardioverter-defibrillator. Circ Cardiovasc Imaging 2009; 2(3): 183-90.
[http://dx.doi.org/10.1161/CIRCIMAGING.108.826529] [PMID: 19808591]

[52] Schmidt A, Azevedo CF, Cheng A, *et al.* Infarct tissue heterogeneity by magnetic resonance imaging identifies enhanced cardiac arrhythmia susceptibility in patients with left ventricular dysfunction. Circulation 2007; 115(15): 2006-14.
[http://dx.doi.org/10.1161/CIRCULATIONAHA.106.653568] [PMID: 17389270]

[53] Abdel-Aty H, Cocker M, Meek C, Tyberg JV, Friedrich MG. Edema as a very early marker for acute myocardial ischemia: a cardiovascular magnetic resonance study. J Am Coll Cardiol 2009; 53(14): 1194-201.
[http://dx.doi.org/10.1016/j.jacc.2008.10.065] [PMID: 19341860]

[54] Cury RC, Shash K, Nagurney JT, *et al.* Cardiac magnetic resonance with T2-weighted imaging improves detection of patients with acute coronary syndrome in the emergency department.

Circulation 2008; 118(8): 837-44.
[http://dx.doi.org/10.1161/CIRCULATIONAHA.107.740597] [PMID: 18678772]

[55]   Wagner A, Mahrholdt H, Holly TA, *et al.* Contrast-enhanced MRI and routine single photon emission computed tomography (SPECT) perfusion imaging for detection of subendocardial myocardial infarcts: an imaging study. Lancet 2003; 361(9355): 374-9.
[http://dx.doi.org/10.1016/S0140-6736(03)12389-6] [PMID: 12573373]

[56]   Casolo G, Minneci S, Manta R, *et al.* Identification of the ischemic etiology of heart failure by cardiovascular magnetic resonance imaging: diagnostic accuracy of late gadolinium enhancement. Am Heart J 2006; 151(1): 101-8.
[http://dx.doi.org/10.1016/j.ahj.2005.03.068] [PMID: 16368300]

[57]   Soriano CJ, Ridocci F, Estornell J, Jimenez J, Martinez V, De Velasco JA. Noninvasive diagnosis of coronary artery disease in patients with heart failure and systolic dysfunction of uncertain etiology, using late gadolinium-enhanced cardiovascular magnetic resonance. J Am Coll Cardiol 2005; 45(5): 743-8.
[http://dx.doi.org/10.1016/j.jacc.2004.11.037] [PMID: 15734620]

[58]   Bekkers SC, Yazdani SK, Virmani R, Waltenberger J. Microvascular obstruction: underlying pathophysiology and clinical diagnosis. J Am Coll Cardiol 2010; 55(16): 1649-60.
[http://dx.doi.org/10.1016/j.jacc.2009.12.037] [PMID: 20394867]

[59]   Nijveldt R, Hofman MB, Hirsch A, *et al.* Assessment of microvascular obstruction and prediction of short-term remodeling after acute myocardial infarction: cardiac MR imaging study. Radiology 2009; 250(2): 363-70.
[http://dx.doi.org/10.1148/radiol.2502080739] [PMID: 19164698]

[60]   Nijveldt R, Beek AM, Hirsch A, *et al.* Functional recovery after acute myocardial infarction: comparison between angiography, electrocardiography, and cardiovascular magnetic resonance measures of microvascular injury. J Am Coll Cardiol 2008; 52(3): 181-9.
[http://dx.doi.org/10.1016/j.jacc.2008.04.006] [PMID: 18617066]

[61]   Wu KC, Zerhouni EA, Judd RM, *et al.* Prognostic significance of microvascular obstruction by magnetic resonance imaging in patients with acute myocardial infarction. Circulation 1998; 97(8): 765-72.
[http://dx.doi.org/10.1161/01.CIR.97.8.765] [PMID: 9498540]

[62]   Ganame J, Messalli G, Dymarkowski S, *et al.* Impact of myocardial haemorrhage on left ventricular function and remodelling in patients with reperfused acute myocardial infarction. Eur Heart J 2009; 30(12): 1440-9.
[http://dx.doi.org/10.1093/eurheartj/ehp093] [PMID: 19346229]

[63]   Aldrovandi A, De Ridder SP, Strohm O, Cocker M, Sandonato R, Friedrich MG. Detection of papillary muscle infarction by late gadolinium enhancement: incremental value of short-inversion time *vs.* standard imaging. Eur Heart J Cardiovasc Imaging 2013; 14(5): 495-9.
[http://dx.doi.org/10.1093/ehjci/jes210] [PMID: 23082008]

[64]   Weinsaft JW, Kim RJ, Ross M, *et al.* Contrast-enhanced anatomic imaging as compared to contrast-enhanced tissue characterization for detection of left ventricular thrombus. JACC Cardiovasc Imaging 2009; 2(8): 969-79.
[http://dx.doi.org/10.1016/j.jcmg.2009.03.017] [PMID: 19679285]

[65]   Kim HW, Farzaneh-Far A, Kim RJ. Cardiovascular magnetic resonance in patients with myocardial infarction: current and emerging applications. J Am Coll Cardiol 2009; 55(1): 1-16.
[http://dx.doi.org/10.1016/j.jacc.2009.06.059] [PMID: 20117357]

[66]   Heatlie GJ, Mohiaddin R. Left ventricular aneurysm: comprehensive assessment of morphology, structure and thrombus using cardiovascular magnetic resonance. Clin Radiol 2005; 60(6): 687-92.
[http://dx.doi.org/10.1016/j.crad.2005.01.007] [PMID: 16038696]

[67]   Nandalur KR, Dwamena BA, Choudhri AF, Nandalur MR, Carlos RC. Diagnostic performance of

stress cardiac magnetic resonance imaging in the detection of coronary artery disease: a meta-analysis. J Am Coll Cardiol 2007; 50(14): 1343-53.
[http://dx.doi.org/10.1016/j.jacc.2007.06.030] [PMID: 17903634]

[68] Greenwood JP, Motwani M, Maredia N, *et al.* Comparison of cardiovascular magnetic resonance and single-photon emission computed tomography in women with suspected coronary artery disease from the Clinical Evaluation of Magnetic Resonance Imaging in Coronary Heart Disease (CE-MARC) Trial. Circulation 2014; 129(10): 1129-38.
[http://dx.doi.org/10.1161/CIRCULATIONAHA.112.000071] [PMID: 24357404]

[69] Nagel E, Klein C, Paetsch I, *et al.* Magnetic resonance perfusion measurements for the noninvasive detection of coronary artery disease. Circulation 2003; 108(4): 432-7.
[http://dx.doi.org/10.1161/01.CIR.0000080915.35024.A9] [PMID: 12860910]

[70] Karamitsos TD, Arnold JR, Pegg TJ, *et al.* Tolerance and safety of adenosine stress perfusion cardiovascular magnetic resonance imaging in patients with severe coronary artery disease. Int J Cardiovasc Imaging 2009; 25(3): 277-83.
[http://dx.doi.org/10.1007/s10554-008-9392-3] [PMID: 19037746]

[71] Wahl A, Paetsch I, Gollesch A, *et al.* Safety and feasibility of high-dose dobutamine-atropine stress cardiovascular magnetic resonance for diagnosis of myocardial ischaemia: experience in 1000 consecutive cases. Eur Heart J 2004; 25(14): 1230-6.
[http://dx.doi.org/10.1016/j.ehj.2003.11.018] [PMID: 15246641]

[72] Wellnhofer E, Olariu A, Klein C, *et al.* Magnetic resonance low-dose dobutamine test is superior to SCAR quantification for the prediction of functional recovery. Circulation 2004; 109(18): 2172-4.
[http://dx.doi.org/10.1161/01.CIR.0000128862.34201.74] [PMID: 15117834]

[73] Gimelli A, Lancellotti P, Badano LP, *et al.* Non-invasive cardiac imaging evaluation of patients with chronic systolic heart failure: a report from the European Association of Cardiovascular Imaging (EACVI). Eur Heart J 2014; 35(48): 3417-25.
[http://dx.doi.org/10.1093/eurheartj/ehu433] [PMID: 25416326]

[74] Kim WY, Danias PG, Stuber M, *et al.* Coronary magnetic resonance angiography for the detection of coronary stenoses. N Engl J Med 2001; 345(26): 1863-9.
[http://dx.doi.org/10.1056/NEJMoa010866] [PMID: 11756576]

[75] Kato S, Kitagawa K, Ishida N, *et al.* Assessment of coronary artery disease using magnetic resonance coronary angiography: a national multicenter trial. J Am Coll Cardiol 2010; 56(12): 983-91.
[http://dx.doi.org/10.1016/j.jacc.2010.01.071] [PMID: 20828652]

[76] Bluemke DA, Achenbach S, Budoff M, *et al.* Noninvasive coronary artery imaging: magnetic resonance angiography and multidetector computed tomography angiography: a scientific statement from the american heart association committee on cardiovascular imaging and intervention of the council on cardiovascular radiology and intervention, and the councils on clinical cardiology and cardiovascular disease in the young. Circulation 2008; 118(5): 586-606.
[http://dx.doi.org/10.1161/CIRCULATIONAHA.108.189695] [PMID: 18586979]

[77] Caforio AL, Mahon NG, Baig MK, *et al.* Prospective familial assessment in dilated cardiomyopathy: cardiac autoantibodies predict disease development in asymptomatic relatives. Circulation 2007; 115(1): 76-83.
[http://dx.doi.org/10.1161/CIRCULATIONAHA.106.641472] [PMID: 17179019]

[78] Roberts WC, Siegel RJ, McManus BM. Idiopathic dilated cardiomyopathy: analysis of 152 necropsy patients. Am J Cardiol 1987; 60(16): 1340-55.
[http://dx.doi.org/10.1016/0002-9149(87)90618-7] [PMID: 3687784]

[79] Bogun FM, Desjardins B, Good E, *et al.* Delayed-enhanced magnetic resonance imaging in nonischemic cardiomyopathy: utility for identifying the ventricular arrhythmia substrate. J Am Coll Cardiol 2009; 53(13): 1138-45.
[http://dx.doi.org/10.1016/j.jacc.2008.11.052] [PMID: 19324259]

[80] Goldberger JJ, Buxton AE, Cain M, *et al.* Risk stratification for arrhythmic sudden cardiac death: identifying the roadblocks. Circulation 2011; 123(21): 2423-30.
[http://dx.doi.org/10.1161/CIRCULATIONAHA.110.959734] [PMID: 21632516]

[81] Stecker EC, Chugh SS. Prediction of sudden cardiac death: next steps in pursuit of effective methodology. J Interv Card Electrophysiol 2011; 31(2): 101-7.
[http://dx.doi.org/10.1007/s10840-010-9535-z] [PMID: 21384153]

[82] Gulati A, Jabbour A, Ismail TF, *et al.* Association of fibrosis with mortality and sudden cardiac death in patients with nonischemic dilated cardiomyopathy. JAMA 2013; 309(9): 896-908.
[http://dx.doi.org/10.1001/jama.2013.1363] [PMID: 23462786]

[83] Moreo A, Ambrosio G, De Chiara B, *et al.* Influence of myocardial fibrosis on left ventricular diastolic function: noninvasive assessment by cardiac magnetic resonance and echo. Circ Cardiovasc Imaging 2009; 2(6): 437-43.
[http://dx.doi.org/10.1161/CIRCIMAGING.108.838367] [PMID: 19920041]

[84] Friedrich MG, Sechtem U, Schulz-Menger J, *et al.* Cardiovascular magnetic resonance in myocarditis: A JACC White Paper. J Am Coll Cardiol 2009; 53(17): 1475-87.
[http://dx.doi.org/10.1016/j.jacc.2009.02.007] [PMID: 19389557]

[85] Friedrich MG, Strohm O, Schulz-Menger J, Marciniak H, Luft FC, Dietz R. Contrast media-enhanced magnetic resonance imaging visualizes myocardial changes in the course of viral myocarditis. Circulation 1998; 97(18): 1802-9.
[http://dx.doi.org/10.1161/01.CIR.97.18.1802] [PMID: 9603535]

[86] Abdel-Aty H, Boyé P, Zagrosek A, *et al.* Diagnostic performance of cardiovascular magnetic resonance in patients with suspected acute myocarditis: comparison of different approaches. J Am Coll Cardiol 2005; 45(11): 1815-22.
[http://dx.doi.org/10.1016/j.jacc.2004.11.069] [PMID: 15936612]

[87] Mahrholdt H, Goedecke C, Wagner A, *et al.* Cardiovascular magnetic resonance assessment of human myocarditis: a comparison to histology and molecular pathology. Circulation 2004; 109(10): 1250-8.
[http://dx.doi.org/10.1161/01.CIR.0000118493.13323.81] [PMID: 14993139]

[88] Murphy RT, Thaman R, Blanes JG, *et al.* Natural history and familial characteristics of isolated left ventricular non-compaction. Eur Heart J 2005; 26(2): 187-92.
[http://dx.doi.org/10.1093/eurheartj/ehi025] [PMID: 15618076]

[89] Jenni R, Oechslin E, Schneider J, Attenhofer Jost C, Kaufmann PA. Echocardiographic and pathoanatomical characteristics of isolated left ventricular non-compaction: a step towards classification as a distinct cardiomyopathy. Heart 2001; 86(6): 666-71.
[http://dx.doi.org/10.1136/heart.86.6.666] [PMID: 11711464]

[90] Kohli SK, Pantazis AA, Shah JS, *et al.* Diagnosis of left-ventricular non-compaction in patients with left-ventricular systolic dysfunction: time for a reappraisal of diagnostic criteria? Eur Heart J 2008; 29(1): 89-95.
[http://dx.doi.org/10.1093/eurheartj/ehm481] [PMID: 17993472]

[91] Gati S, Rajani R, Carr-White GS, Chambers JB. Adult left ventricular noncompaction: reappraisal of current diagnostic imaging modalities. JACC Cardiovasc Imaging 2014; 7(12): 1266-75.
[http://dx.doi.org/10.1016/j.jcmg.2014.09.005] [PMID: 25496545]

[92] Petersen SE, Selvanayagam JB, Wiesmann F, *et al.* Left ventricular non-compaction: insights from cardiovascular magnetic resonance imaging. J Am Coll Cardiol 2005; 46(1): 101-5.
[http://dx.doi.org/10.1016/j.jacc.2005.03.045] [PMID: 15992642]

[93] Stacey RB, Andersen MM, St Clair M, Hundley WG, Thohan V. Comparison of systolic and diastolic criteria for isolated LV noncompaction in CMR. JACC Cardiovasc Imaging 2013; 6(9): 931-40.
[http://dx.doi.org/10.1016/j.jcmg.2013.01.014] [PMID: 23769489]

[94] Jacquier A, Thuny F, Jop B, *et al.* Measurement of trabeculated left ventricular mass using cardiac

magnetic resonance imaging in the diagnosis of left ventricular non-compaction. Eur Heart J 2010; 31(9): 1098-104.
[http://dx.doi.org/10.1093/eurheartj/ehp595] [PMID: 20089517]

[95] Wan J, Zhao S, Cheng H, *et al.* Varied distributions of late gadolinium enhancement found among patients meeting cardiovascular magnetic resonance criteria for isolated left ventricular non-compaction. J Cardiovasc Magn Reson 2013; 15: 20.
[http://dx.doi.org/10.1186/1532-429X-15-20] [PMID: 23421977]

[96] Nucifora G, Aquaro GD, Pingitore A, Masci PG, Lombardi M. Myocardial fibrosis in isolated left ventricular non-compaction and its relation to disease severity. Eur J Heart Fail 2011; 13(2): 170-6.
[http://dx.doi.org/10.1093/eurjhf/hfq222] [PMID: 21208941]

[97] Stacey RB, Andersen M, Haag J, *et al.* Right ventricular morphology and systolic function in left ventricular noncompaction cardiomyopathy. Am J Cardiol 2014; 113(6): 1018-23.
[http://dx.doi.org/10.1016/j.amjcard.2013.12.008] [PMID: 24462071]

[98] Silverman KJ, Hutchins GM, Bulkley BH. Cardiac sarcoid: a clinicopathologic study of 84 unselected patients with systemic sarcoidosis. Circulation 1978; 58(6): 1204-11.
[http://dx.doi.org/10.1161/01.CIR.58.6.1204] [PMID: 709777]

[99] Doughan AR, Williams BR. Cardiac sarcoidosis. Heart 2006; 92(2): 282-8.
[http://dx.doi.org/10.1136/hrt.2005.080481] [PMID: 16415205]

[100] Roberts WC, McAllister HA Jr, Ferrans VJ. Sarcoidosis of the heart. A clinicopathologic study of 35 necropsy patients (group 1) and review of 78 previously described necropsy patients (group 11). Am J Med 1977; 63(1): 86-108.
[http://dx.doi.org/10.1016/0002-9343(77)90121-8] [PMID: 327806]

[101] Tadamura E, Yamamuro M, Kubo S, *et al.* Effectiveness of delayed enhanced MRI for identification of cardiac sarcoidosis: comparison with radionuclide imaging. AJR Am J Roentgenol 2005; 185(1): 110-5.
[http://dx.doi.org/10.2214/ajr.185.1.01850110] [PMID: 15972409]

[102] Radulescu B, Imperiale A, Germain P, Ohlmann P. Severe ventricular arrhythmias in a patient with cardiac sarcoidosis: insights from MRI and PET imaging and importance of early corticosteroid therapy. Eur Heart J 2010; 31(4): 400.
[http://dx.doi.org/10.1093/eurheartj/ehp456] [PMID: 19854726]

[103] Smedema JP, Snoep G, van Kroonenburgh MP, *et al.* Evaluation of the accuracy of gadolinium-enhanced cardiovascular magnetic resonance in the diagnosis of cardiac sarcoidosis. J Am Coll Cardiol 2005; 45(10): 1683-90.
[http://dx.doi.org/10.1016/j.jacc.2005.01.047] [PMID: 15893188]

[104] Smedema JP, Truter R, de Klerk PA, Zaaiman L, White L, Doubell AF. Cardiac sarcoidosis evaluated with gadolinium-enhanced magnetic resonance and contrast-enhanced 64-slice computed tomography. Int J Cardiol 2006; 112(2): 261-3.
[http://dx.doi.org/10.1016/j.ijcard.2005.07.059] [PMID: 16257460]

[105] Yared K, Johri AM, Soni AV, *et al.* Cardiac sarcoidosis imitating arrhythmogenic right ventricular dysplasia. Circulation 2008; 118(7): e113-5.
[http://dx.doi.org/10.1161/CIRCULATIONAHA.107.755215] [PMID: 18695196]

[106] Soejima K, Yada H. The work-up and management of patients with apparent or subclinical cardiac sarcoidosis: with emphasis on the associated heart rhythm abnormalities. J Cardiovasc Electrophysiol 2009; 20(5): 578-83.
[http://dx.doi.org/10.1111/j.1540-8167.2008.01417.x] [PMID: 19175448]

[107] Patel MR, Cawley PJ, Heitner JF, *et al.* Detection of myocardial damage in patients with sarcoidosis. Circulation 2009; 120(20): 1969-77.
[http://dx.doi.org/10.1161/CIRCULATIONAHA.109.851352] [PMID: 19884472]

[108] Schulz-Menger J, Wassmuth R, Abdel-Aty H, *et al.* Patterns of myocardial inflammation and scarring in sarcoidosis as assessed by cardiovascular magnetic resonance. Heart 2006; 92(3): 399-400.
[http://dx.doi.org/10.1136/hrt.2004.058016] [PMID: 16501203]

[109] Gujja P, Rosing DR, Tripodi DJ, Shizukuda Y. Iron overload cardiomyopathy: better understanding of an increasing disorder. J Am Coll Cardiol 2010; 56(13): 1001-12.
[http://dx.doi.org/10.1016/j.jacc.2010.03.083] [PMID: 20846597]

[110] Carpenter JP, He T, Kirk P, *et al.* On T2* magnetic resonance and cardiac iron. Circulation 2011; 123(14): 1519-28.
[http://dx.doi.org/10.1161/CIRCULATIONAHA.110.007641] [PMID: 21444881]

[111] Anderson LJ, Holden S, Davis B, *et al.* Cardiovascular T2-star (T2*) magnetic resonance for the early diagnosis of myocardial iron overload. Eur Heart J 2001; 22(23): 2171-9.
[http://dx.doi.org/10.1053/euhj.2001.2822] [PMID: 11913479]

[112] Marsella M, Borgna-Pignatti C, Meloni A, *et al.* Cardiac iron and cardiac disease in males and females with transfusion-dependent thalassemia major: a T2* magnetic resonance imaging study. Haematologica 2011; 96(4): 515-20.
[http://dx.doi.org/10.3324/haematol.2010.025510] [PMID: 21228034]

[113] Kirk P, Roughton M, Porter JB, *et al.* Cardiac T2* magnetic resonance for prediction of cardiac complications in thalassemia major. Circulation 2009; 120(20): 1961-8.
[http://dx.doi.org/10.1161/CIRCULATIONAHA.109.874487] [PMID: 19801505]

[114] Modell B, Khan M, Darlison M, Westwood MA, Ingram D, Pennell DJ. Improved survival of thalassaemia major in the UK and relation to T2* cardiovascular magnetic resonance. J Cardiovasc Magn Reson 2008; 10: 42.
[http://dx.doi.org/10.1186/1532-429X-10-42] [PMID: 18817553]

[115] Bybee KA, Kara T, Prasad A, *et al.* Systematic review: transient left ventricular apical ballooning: a syndrome that mimics ST-segment elevation myocardial infarction. Ann Intern Med 2004; 141(11): 858-65.
[http://dx.doi.org/10.7326/0003-4819-141-11-200412070-00010] [PMID: 15583228]

[116] Tsuchihashi K, Ueshima K, Uchida T, *et al.* Transient left ventricular apical ballooning without coronary artery stenosis: a novel heart syndrome mimicking acute myocardial infarction. Angina Pectoris-Myocardial Infarction Investigations in Japan. J Am Coll Cardiol 2001; 38(1): 11-8.
[http://dx.doi.org/10.1016/S0735-1097(01)01316-X] [PMID: 11451258]

[117] Eitel I, von Knobelsdorff-Brenkenhoff F, Bernhardt P, *et al.* Clinical characteristics and cardiovascular magnetic resonance findings in stress (takotsubo) cardiomyopathy. JAMA 2011; 306(3): 277-86.
[http://dx.doi.org/10.1001/jama.2011.992] [PMID: 21771988]

[118] Owan TE, Hodge DO, Herges RM, Jacobsen SJ, Roger VL, Redfield MM. Trends in prevalence and outcome of heart failure with preserved ejection fraction. N Engl J Med 2006; 355(3): 251-9.
[http://dx.doi.org/10.1056/NEJMoa052256] [PMID: 16855265]

[119] Paulus WJ, Tschöpe C, Sanderson JE, *et al.* How to diagnose diastolic heart failure: a consensus statement on the diagnosis of heart failure with normal left ventricular ejection fraction by the Heart Failure and Echocardiography Associations of the European Society of Cardiology. Eur Heart J 2007; 28(20): 2539-50.
[http://dx.doi.org/10.1093/eurheartj/ehm037] [PMID: 17428822]

[120] Katz J, Milliken MC, Stray-Gundersen J, *et al.* Estimation of human myocardial mass with MR imaging. Radiology 1988; 169(2): 495-8.
[http://dx.doi.org/10.1148/radiology.169.2.2971985] [PMID: 2971985]

[121] Grothues F, Smith GC, Moon JC, *et al.* Comparison of interstudy reproducibility of cardiovascular magnetic resonance with two-dimensional echocardiography in normal subjects and in patients with heart failure or left ventricular hypertrophy. Am J Cardiol 2002; 90(1): 29-34.

[http://dx.doi.org/10.1016/S0002-9149(02)02381-0] [PMID: 12088775]

[122] Kudelka AM, Turner DA, Liebson PR, Macioch JE, Wang JZ, Barron JT. Comparison of cine magnetic resonance imaging and Doppler echocardiography for evaluation of left ventricular diastolic function. Am J Cardiol 1997; 80(3): 384-6.
[http://dx.doi.org/10.1016/S0002-9149(97)00375-5] [PMID: 9264448]

[123] Leong DP, De Pasquale CG, Selvanayagam JB. Heart failure with normal ejection fraction: the complementary roles of echocardiography and CMR imaging. JACC Cardiovasc Imaging 2010; 3(4): 409-20.
[http://dx.doi.org/10.1016/j.jcmg.2009.12.011] [PMID: 20394903]

[124] Maron BJ. Hypertrophic cardiomyopathy: a systematic review. JAMA 2002; 287(10): 1308-20.
[http://dx.doi.org/10.1001/jama.287.10.1308] [PMID: 11886323]

[125] Pons-Lladó G, Carreras F, Borrás X, Palmer J, Llauger J, Bayés de Luna A. Comparison of morphologic assessment of hypertrophic cardiomyopathy by magnetic resonance *versus* echocardiographic imaging. Am J Cardiol 1997; 79(12): 1651-6.
[http://dx.doi.org/10.1016/S0002-9149(97)00216-6] [PMID: 9202357]

[126] Rickers C, Wilke NM, Jerosch-Herold M, *et al*. Utility of cardiac magnetic resonance imaging in the diagnosis of hypertrophic cardiomyopathy. Circulation 2005; 112(6): 855-61.
[http://dx.doi.org/10.1161/CIRCULATIONAHA.104.507723] [PMID: 16087809]

[127] Moon JC, Fisher NG, McKenna WJ, Pennell DJ. Detection of apical hypertrophic cardiomyopathy by cardiovascular magnetic resonance in patients with non-diagnostic echocardiography. Heart 2004; 90(6): 645-9.
[http://dx.doi.org/10.1136/hrt.2003.014969] [PMID: 15145868]

[128] Olivotto I, Maron MS, Autore C, *et al*. Assessment and significance of left ventricular mass by cardiovascular magnetic resonance in hypertrophic cardiomyopathy. J Am Coll Cardiol 2008; 52(7): 559-66.
[http://dx.doi.org/10.1016/j.jacc.2008.04.047] [PMID: 18687251]

[129] Maron MS, Finley JJ, Bos JM, *et al*. Prevalence, clinical significance, and natural history of left ventricular apical aneurysms in hypertrophic cardiomyopathy. Circulation 2008; 118(15): 1541-9.
[http://dx.doi.org/10.1161/CIRCULATIONAHA.108.781401] [PMID: 18809796]

[130] Spirito P, Bellone P, Harris KM, Bernabo P, Bruzzi P, Maron BJ. Magnitude of left ventricular hypertrophy and risk of sudden death in hypertrophic cardiomyopathy. N Engl J Med 2000; 342(24): 1778-85.
[http://dx.doi.org/10.1056/NEJM200006153422403] [PMID: 10853000]

[131] Kwon DH, Setser RM, Thamilarasan M, *et al*. Abnormal papillary muscle morphology is independently associated with increased left ventricular outflow tract obstruction in hypertrophic cardiomyopathy. Heart 2008; 94(10): 1295-301.
[http://dx.doi.org/10.1136/hrt.2007.118018] [PMID: 17690158]

[132] Rudolph A, Abdel-Aty H, Bohl S, *et al*. Noninvasive detection of fibrosis applying contrast-enhanced cardiac magnetic resonance in different forms of left ventricular hypertrophy relation to remodeling. J Am Coll Cardiol 2009; 53(3): 284-91.
[http://dx.doi.org/10.1016/j.jacc.2008.08.064] [PMID: 19147047]

[133] Chan RH, Maron BJ, Olivotto I, *et al*. Prognostic value of quantitative contrast-enhanced cardiovascular magnetic resonance for the evaluation of sudden death risk in patients with hypertrophic cardiomyopathy. Circulation 2014; 130(6): 484-95.
[http://dx.doi.org/10.1161/CIRCULATIONAHA.113.007094] [PMID: 25092278]

[134] Adabag AS, Maron BJ, Appelbaum E, *et al*. Occurrence and frequency of arrhythmias in hypertrophic cardiomyopathy in relation to delayed enhancement on cardiovascular magnetic resonance. J Am Coll Cardiol 2008; 51(14): 1369-74.
[http://dx.doi.org/10.1016/j.jacc.2007.11.071] [PMID: 18387438]

[135] Clarke JT. Narrative review: Fabry disease. Ann Intern Med 2007; 146(6): 425-33.
[http://dx.doi.org/10.7326/0003-4819-146-6-200703200-00007] [PMID: 17371887]

[136] Sachdev B, Takenaka T, Teraguchi H, *et al.* Prevalence of Anderson-Fabry disease in male patients with late onset hypertrophic cardiomyopathy. Circulation 2002; 105(12): 1407-11.
[http://dx.doi.org/10.1161/01.CIR.0000012626.81324.38] [PMID: 11914245]

[137] Frustaci A, Chimenti C, Ricci R, *et al.* Improvement in cardiac function in the cardiac variant of Fabry's disease with galactose-infusion therapy. N Engl J Med 2001; 345(1): 25-32.
[http://dx.doi.org/10.1056/NEJM200107053450104] [PMID: 11439944]

[138] Moon JC, Sheppard M, Reed E, Lee P, Elliott PM, Pennell DJ. The histological basis of late gadolinium enhancement cardiovascular magnetic resonance in a patient with Anderson-Fabry disease. J Cardiovasc Magn Reson 2006; 8(3): 479-82.
[http://dx.doi.org/10.1080/10976640600605002] [PMID: 16755835]

[139] De Cobelli F, Esposito A, Belloni E, *et al.* Delayed-enhanced cardiac MRI for differentiation of Fabry's disease from symmetric hypertrophic cardiomyopathy. AJR Am J Roentgenol 2009; 192(3)W97-102
[http://dx.doi.org/10.2214/AJR.08.1201] [PMID: 19234246]

[140] Moon JC, Sachdev B, Elkington AG, *et al.* Gadolinium enhanced cardiovascular magnetic resonance in Anderson-Fabry disease. Evidence for a disease specific abnormality of the myocardial interstitium. Eur Heart J 2003; 24(23): 2151-5.
[http://dx.doi.org/10.1016/j.ehj.2003.09.017] [PMID: 14643276]

[141] Selvanayagam JB, Hawkins PN, Paul B, Myerson SG, Neubauer S. Evaluation and management of the cardiac amyloidosis. J Am Coll Cardiol 2007; 50(22): 2101-10.
[http://dx.doi.org/10.1016/j.jacc.2007.08.028] [PMID: 18036445]

[142] Falk RH, Skinner M. The systemic amyloidoses: an overview. Adv Intern Med 2000; 45: 107-37.
[PMID: 10635047]

[143] Vogelsberg H, Mahrholdt H, Deluigi CC, *et al.* Cardiovascular magnetic resonance in clinically suspected cardiac amyloidosis: noninvasive imaging compared to endomyocardial biopsy. J Am Coll Cardiol 2008; 51(10): 1022-30.
[http://dx.doi.org/10.1016/j.jacc.2007.10.049] [PMID: 18325442]

[144] Maceira AM, Joshi J, Prasad SK, *et al.* Cardiovascular magnetic resonance in cardiac amyloidosis. Circulation 2005; 111(2): 186-93.
[http://dx.doi.org/10.1161/01.CIR.0000152819.97857.9D] [PMID: 15630027]

[145] Cheng AS, Banning AP, Mitchell AR, Neubauer S, Selvanayagam JB. Cardiac changes in systemic amyloidosis: visualisation by magnetic resonance imaging. Int J Cardiol 2006; 113(1): E21-3.
[http://dx.doi.org/10.1016/j.ijcard.2006.07.107] [PMID: 17049635]

[146] Ruberg FL, Appelbaum E, Davidoff R, *et al.* Diagnostic and prognostic utility of cardiovascular magnetic resonance imaging in light-chain cardiac amyloidosis. Am J Cardiol 2009; 103(4): 544-9.
[http://dx.doi.org/10.1016/j.amjcard.2008.09.105] [PMID: 19195518]

[147] Maceira AM, Prasad SK, Hawkins PN, Roughton M, Pennell DJ. Cardiovascular magnetic resonance and prognosis in cardiac amyloidosis. J Cardiovasc Magn Reson 2008; 10: 54.
[http://dx.doi.org/10.1186/1532-429X-10-54] [PMID: 19032744]

[148] Hulot JS, Jouven X, Empana JP, Frank R, Fontaine G. Natural history and risk stratification of arrhythmogenic right ventricular dysplasia/cardiomyopathy. Circulation 2004; 110(14): 1879-84.
[http://dx.doi.org/10.1161/01.CIR.0000143375.93288.82] [PMID: 15451782]

[149] Gemayel C, Pelliccia A, Thompson PD. Arrhythmogenic right ventricular cardiomyopathy. J Am Coll Cardiol 2001; 38(7): 1773-81.
[http://dx.doi.org/10.1016/S0735-1097(01)01654-0] [PMID: 11738273]

[150] Sen-Chowdhry S, Lowe MD, Sporton SC, McKenna WJ. Arrhythmogenic right ventricular cardiomyopathy: clinical presentation, diagnosis, and management. Am J Med 2004; 117(9): 685-95.
[http://dx.doi.org/10.1016/j.amjmed.2004.04.028] [PMID: 15501207]

[151] Tandri H, Saranathan M, Rodriguez ER, *et al.* Noninvasive detection of myocardial fibrosis in arrhythmogenic right ventricular cardiomyopathy using delayed-enhancement magnetic resonance imaging. J Am Coll Cardiol 2005; 45(1): 98-103.
[http://dx.doi.org/10.1016/j.jacc.2004.09.053] [PMID: 15629382]

[152] Marcus FI, McKenna WJ, Sherrill D, *et al.* Diagnosis of arrhythmogenic right ventricular cardiomyopathy/dysplasia: proposed modification of the task force criteria. Circulation 2010; 121(13): 1533-41.
[http://dx.doi.org/10.1161/CIRCULATIONAHA.108.840827] [PMID: 20172911]

[153] Tandri H, Castillo E, Ferrari VA, *et al.* Magnetic resonance imaging of arrhythmogenic right ventricular dysplasia: sensitivity, specificity, and observer variability of fat detection *versus* functional analysis of the right ventricle. J Am Coll Cardiol 2006; 48(11): 2277-84.
[http://dx.doi.org/10.1016/j.jacc.2006.07.051] [PMID: 17161260]

[154] Hunold P, Wieneke H, Bruder O, *et al.* Late enhancement: a new feature in MRI of arrhythmogenic right ventricular cardiomyopathy? J Cardiovasc Magn Reson 2005; 7(4): 649-55.
[http://dx.doi.org/10.1081/JCMR-200065608] [PMID: 16136854]

[155] Masui T, Finck S, Higgins CB. Constrictive pericarditis and restrictive cardiomyopathy: evaluation with MR imaging. Radiology 1992; 182(2): 369-73.
[http://dx.doi.org/10.1148/radiology.182.2.1732952] [PMID: 1732952]

[156] Wang ZJ, Reddy GP, Gotway MB, Yeh BM, Hetts SW, Higgins CBCT. CT and MR imaging of pericardial disease. Radiographics 2003; 23(Spec No): S167-80.
[http://dx.doi.org/10.1148/rg.23si035504] [PMID: 14557510]

[157] Francone M, Dymarkowski S, Kalantzi M, Rademakers FE, Bogaert J. Assessment of ventricular coupling with real-time cine MRI and its value to differentiate constrictive pericarditis from restrictive cardiomyopathy. Eur Radiol 2006; 16(4): 944-51.
[http://dx.doi.org/10.1007/s00330-005-0009-0] [PMID: 16228208]

[158] White JA, Yee R, Yuan X, *et al.* Delayed enhancement magnetic resonance imaging predicts response to cardiac resynchronization therapy in patients with intraventricular dyssynchrony. J Am Coll Cardiol 2006; 48(10): 1953-60.
[http://dx.doi.org/10.1016/j.jacc.2006.07.046] [PMID: 17112984]

[159] Ypenburg C, Schalij MJ, Bleeker GB, *et al.* Impact of viability and scar tissue on response to cardiac resynchronization therapy in ischaemic heart failure patients. Eur Heart J 2007; 28(1): 33-41.
[http://dx.doi.org/10.1093/eurheartj/ehl379] [PMID: 17121757]

[160] Reuter S, Garrigue S, Barold SS, *et al.* Comparison of characteristics in responders *versus* nonresponders with biventricular pacing for drug-resistant congestive heart failure. Am J Cardiol 2002; 89(3): 346-50.
[http://dx.doi.org/10.1016/S0002-9149(01)02240-8] [PMID: 11809441]

[161] Bleeker GB, Kaandorp TA, Lamb HJ, *et al.* Effect of posterolateral scar tissue on clinical and echocardiographic improvement after cardiac resynchronization therapy. Circulation 2006; 113(7): 969-76.
[http://dx.doi.org/10.1161/CIRCULATIONAHA.105.543678] [PMID: 16476852]

[162] Usman AA, Taimen K, Wasielewski M, *et al.* Cardiac magnetic resonance T2 mapping in the monitoring and follow-up of acute cardiac transplant rejection: a pilot study. Circ Cardiovasc Imaging 2012; 5(6): 782-90.
[http://dx.doi.org/10.1161/CIRCIMAGING.111.971101] [PMID: 23071145]

[163] Marwick TH, Schwaiger M. The future of cardiovascular imaging in the diagnosis and management of

heart failure, part 2: clinical applications. Circ Cardiovasc Imaging 2008; 1(2): 162-70.
[http://dx.doi.org/10.1161/CIRCIMAGING.108.811109] [PMID: 19808534]

[164] Kramer CM, Chandrashekhar Y, Narula J. T1 mapping by CMR in cardiomyopathy: a noninvasive myocardial biopsy? JACC Cardiovasc Imaging 2013; 6(4): 532-4.
[http://dx.doi.org/10.1016/j.jcmg.2013.02.002] [PMID: 23579019]

[165] Sibley CT, Noureldin RA, Gai N, *et al.* T1 Mapping in cardiomyopathy at cardiac MR: comparison with endomyocardial biopsy. Radiology 2012; 265(3): 724-32.
[http://dx.doi.org/10.1148/radiol.12112721] [PMID: 23091172]

[166] Moon JC, Messroghli DR, Kellman P, *et al.* Myocardial T1 mapping and extracellular volume quantification: a Society for Cardiovascular Magnetic Resonance (SCMR) and CMR Working Group of the European Society of Cardiology consensus statement. J Cardiovasc Magn Reson 2013; 15: 92.
[http://dx.doi.org/10.1186/1532-429X-15-92] [PMID: 24124732]

[167] Mascherbauer J, Marzluf BA, Tufaro C, *et al.* Cardiac magnetic resonance postcontrast T1 time is associated with outcome in patients with heart failure and preserved ejection fraction. Circ Cardiovasc Imaging 2013; 6(6): 1056-65.
[http://dx.doi.org/10.1161/CIRCIMAGING.113.000633] [PMID: 24036385]

[168] Puntmann VO, Voigt T, Chen Z, *et al.* Native T1 mapping in differentiation of normal myocardium from diffuse disease in hypertrophic and dilated cardiomyopathy. JACC Cardiovasc Imaging 2013; 6(4): 475-84.
[http://dx.doi.org/10.1016/j.jcmg.2012.08.019] [PMID: 23498674]

[169] Frydrychowicz A, Berger A, Russe MF, *et al.* Time-resolved magnetic resonance angiography and flow-sensitive 4-dimensional magnetic resonance imaging at 3 Tesla for blood flow and wall shear stress analysis. J Thorac Cardiovasc Surg 2008; 136(2): 400-7.
[http://dx.doi.org/10.1016/j.jtcvs.2008.02.062] [PMID: 18692649]

[170] Meierhofer C, Schneider EP, Lyko C, *et al.* Wall shear stress and flow patterns in the ascending aorta in patients with bicuspid aortic valves differ significantly from tricuspid aortic valves: a prospective study. Eur Heart J Cardiovasc Imaging 2013; 14(8): 797-804.
[http://dx.doi.org/10.1093/ehjci/jes273] [PMID: 23230276]

[171] Scollan DF, Holmes A, Winslow R, Forder J. Histological validation of myocardial microstructure obtained from diffusion tensor magnetic resonance imaging. Am J Physiol 1998; 275(6): H2308-18.
[PMID: 9843833]

[172] Budoff MJ, Dowe D, Jollis JG, *et al.* Diagnostic performance of 64-multidetector row coronary computed tomographic angiography for evaluation of coronary artery stenosis in individuals without known coronary artery disease: results from the prospective multicenter ACCURACY (Assessment by Coronary Computed Tomographic Angiography of Individuals Undergoing Invasive Coronary Angiography) trial. J Am Coll Cardiol 2008; 52(21): 1724-32.
[http://dx.doi.org/10.1016/j.jacc.2008.07.031] [PMID: 19007693]

[173] Miller JM, Rochitte CE, Dewey M, *et al.* Diagnostic performance of coronary angiography by 64-row CT. N Engl J Med 2008; 359(22): 2324-36.
[http://dx.doi.org/10.1056/NEJMoa0806576] [PMID: 19038879]

[174] Ropers D, Rixe J, Anders K, *et al.* Usefulness of multidetector row spiral computed tomography with 64- x 0.6-mm collimation and 330-ms rotation for the noninvasive detection of significant coronary artery stenoses. Am J Cardiol 2006; 97(3): 343-8.
[http://dx.doi.org/10.1016/j.amjcard.2005.08.050] [PMID: 16442393]

[175] Earls JP, Berman EL, Urban BA, *et al.* Prospectively gated transverse coronary CT angiography *versus* retrospectively gated helical technique: improved image quality and reduced radiation dose. Radiology 2008; 246(3): 742-53.
[http://dx.doi.org/10.1148/radiol.2463070989] [PMID: 18195386]

[176] Agatston AS, Janowitz WR, Hildner FJ, Zusmer NR, Viamonte M Jr, Detrano R. Quantification of

coronary artery calcium using ultrafast computed tomography. J Am Coll Cardiol 1990; 15(4): 827-32.
[http://dx.doi.org/10.1016/0735-1097(90)90282-T] [PMID: 2407762]

[177]   Bhatia RS, Tu JV, Lee DS, *et al.* Outcome of heart failure with preserved ejection fraction in a
        population-based study. N Engl J Med 2006; 355(3): 260-9.
        [http://dx.doi.org/10.1056/NEJMoa051530] [PMID: 16855266]

[178]   Moscariello A, Takx RA, Schoepf UJ, *et al.* Coronary CT angiography: image quality, diagnostic
        accuracy, and potential for radiation dose reduction using a novel iterative image reconstruction
        technique-comparison with traditional filtered back projection. Eur Radiol 2011; 21(10): 2130-8.
        [http://dx.doi.org/10.1007/s00330-011-2164-9] [PMID: 21611758]

[179]   Schuhbaeck A, Achenbach S, Layritz C, *et al.* Image quality of ultra-low radiation exposure coronary
        CT angiography with an effective dose <0.1 mSv using high-pitch spiral acquisition and raw data-
        based iterative reconstruction. Eur Radiol 2013; 23(3): 597-606.
        [http://dx.doi.org/10.1007/s00330-012-2656-2] [PMID: 22983283]

[180]   Budoff MJ, Georgiou D, Brody A, *et al.* Ultrafast computed tomography as a diagnostic modality in
        the detection of coronary artery disease: a multicenter study. Circulation 1996; 93(5): 898-904.
        [http://dx.doi.org/10.1161/01.CIR.93.5.898] [PMID: 8598080]

[181]   Haberl R, Becker A, Leber A, *et al.* Correlation of coronary calcification and angiographically
        documented stenoses in patients with suspected coronary artery disease: results of 1,764 patients. J Am
        Coll Cardiol 2001; 37(2): 451-7.
        [http://dx.doi.org/10.1016/S0735-1097(00)01119-0] [PMID: 11216962]

[182]   Nasir K, Michos ED, Blumenthal RS, Raggi P. Detection of high-risk young adults and women by
        coronary calcium and National Cholesterol Education Program Panel III guidelines. J Am Coll Cardiol
        2005; 46(10): 1931-6.
        [http://dx.doi.org/10.1016/j.jacc.2005.07.052] [PMID: 16286182]

[183]   Budoff MJ, Shavelle DM, Lamont DH, *et al.* Usefulness of electron beam computed tomography
        scanning for distinguishing ischemic from nonischemic cardiomyopathy. J Am Coll Cardiol 1998;
        32(5): 1173-8.
        [http://dx.doi.org/10.1016/S0735-1097(98)00387-8] [PMID: 9809922]

[184]   Le T, Ko JY, Kim HT, Akinwale P, Budoff MJ. Comparison of echocardiography and electron beam
        tomography in differentiating the etiology of heart failure. Clin Cardiol 2000; 23(6): 417-20.
        [http://dx.doi.org/10.1002/clc.4960230608] [PMID: 10875031]

[185]   Leening MJ, Elias-Smale SE, Kavousi M, *et al.* Coronary calcification and the risk of heart failure in
        the elderly: the Rotterdam Study. JACC Cardiovasc Imaging 2012; 5(9): 874-80.
        [http://dx.doi.org/10.1016/j.jcmg.2012.03.016] [PMID: 22974798]

[186]   Meijboom WB, Meijs MF, Schuijf JD, *et al.* Diagnostic accuracy of 64-slice computed tomography
        coronary angiography: a prospective, multicenter, multivendor study. J Am Coll Cardiol 2008; 52(25):
        2135-44.
        [http://dx.doi.org/10.1016/j.jacc.2008.08.058] [PMID: 19095130]

[187]   Ghostine S, Caussin C, Habis M, *et al.* Non-invasive diagnosis of ischaemic heart failure using 64-
        slice computed tomography. Eur Heart J 2008; 29(17): 2133-40.
        [http://dx.doi.org/10.1093/eurheartj/ehn072] [PMID: 18385120]

[188]   Andreini D, Pontone G, Pepi M, *et al.* Diagnostic accuracy of multidetector computed tomography
        coronary angiography in patients with dilated cardiomyopathy. J Am Coll Cardiol 2007; 49(20): 2044-
        50.
        [http://dx.doi.org/10.1016/j.jacc.2007.01.086] [PMID: 17512361]

[189]   Koo BK, Erglis A, Doh JH, *et al.* Diagnosis of ischemia-causing coronary stenoses by noninvasive
        fractional flow reserve computed from coronary computed tomographic angiograms. Results from the
        prospective multicenter DISCOVER-FLOW (Diagnosis of Ischemia-Causing Stenoses Obtained Via
        Noninvasive Fractional Flow Reserve) study. J Am Coll Cardiol 2011; 58(19): 1989-97.

[http://dx.doi.org/10.1016/j.jacc.2011.06.066] [PMID: 22032711]

[190]   Min JK, Leipsic J, Pencina MJ, *et al.* Diagnostic accuracy of fractional flow reserve from anatomic CT angiography. JAMA 2012; 308(12): 1237-45.
[http://dx.doi.org/10.1001/2012.jama.11274] [PMID: 22922562]

[191]   Bamberg F, Becker A, Schwarz F, *et al.* Detection of hemodynamically significant coronary artery stenosis: incremental diagnostic value of dynamic CT-based myocardial perfusion imaging. Radiology 2011; 260(3): 689-98.
[http://dx.doi.org/10.1148/radiol.11110638] [PMID: 21846761]

[192]   Patel MR, White RD, Abbara S, *et al.* 2013 ACCF/ACR/ASE/ASNC/SCCT/SCMR appropriate utilization of cardiovascular imaging in heart failure: a joint report of the American College of Radiology Appropriateness Criteria Committee and the American College of Cardiology Foundation Appropriate Use Criteria Task Force. J Am Coll Cardiol 2013; 61(21): 2207-31.
[http://dx.doi.org/10.1016/j.jacc.2013.02.005] [PMID: 23500216]

[193]   Sidhu MS, Uthamalingam S, Ahmed W, *et al.* Defining left ventricular noncompaction using cardiac computed tomography. J Thorac Imaging 2014; 29(1): 60-6.
[http://dx.doi.org/10.1097/RTI.0b013e31828e9b3d] [PMID: 23689383]

[194]   Gopal A, Pal R, Karlsberg RP, Budoff MJ. Left ventricular pseudoaneurysm by cardiac CT angiography. J Invasive Cardiol 2008; 20(7): 370-1.
[PMID: 18599899]

[195]   Rabkin I, Ovtchinnikov V, Judin A. Computed tomographic evaluation of morphological and functional condition of left ventricle in heart aneurysm. Eur J Radiol 1986; 6(1): 15-20.
[PMID: 3699032]

[196]   Raman SV, Shah M, McCarthy B, Garcia A, Ferketich AK. Multi-detector row cardiac computed tomography accurately quantifies right and left ventricular size and function compared with cardiac magnetic resonance. Am Heart J 2006; 151(3): 736-44.
[http://dx.doi.org/10.1016/j.ahj.2005.04.029] [PMID: 16504643]

[197]   Schroeder J, Peterschroeder A, Vaske B, *et al.* Cardiac volumetry in patients with heart failure and reduced ejection fraction: a comparative study correlating multi-slice computed tomography and magnetic resonance tomography. Reasons for intermodal disagreement. Clin Res Cardiol 2009; 98(11): 739-47.
[http://dx.doi.org/10.1007/s00392-009-0074-5] [PMID: 19771459]

[198]   Burianová L, Riedlbauchová L, Lefflerová K, *et al.* Assessment of left ventricular function in non-dilated and dilated hearts: comparison of contrast-enhanced 2-dimensional echocardiography with multi-detector row CT angiography. Acta Cardiol 2009; 64(6): 787-94.
[http://dx.doi.org/10.2143/AC.64.6.2044744] [PMID: 20128156]

[199]   Yang Y, Yam Y, Chen L, Aljizeeri A, Aliyary Ghraboghly S, Al-Harbi I, *et al.* Assessment of left ventricular ejection fraction using low radiation dose computed tomography. J Nucl Cardiol 2015.
[PMID: 26002814]

[200]   Bittencourt MS, Achenbach S, Marwan M, *et al.* Left ventricular thrombus attenuation characterization in cardiac computed tomography angiography. J Cardiovasc Comput Tomogr 2012; 6(2): 121-6.
[http://dx.doi.org/10.1016/j.jcct.2011.12.006] [PMID: 22342878]

[201]   Hur J, Kim YJ, Lee HJ, *et al.* Left atrial appendage thrombi in stroke patients: detection with two-phase cardiac CT angiography *versus* transesophageal echocardiography. Radiology 2009; 251(3): 683-90.
[http://dx.doi.org/10.1148/radiol.2513090794] [PMID: 19366905]

[202]   Martinez MW, Kirsch J, Williamson EE, *et al.* Utility of nongated multidetector computed tomography for detection of left atrial thrombus in patients undergoing catheter ablation of atrial fibrillation. JACC Cardiovasc Imaging 2009; 2(1): 69-76.

[http://dx.doi.org/10.1016/j.jcmg.2008.09.011] [PMID: 19356536]

[203] Lardo AC, Cordeiro MA, Silva C, *et al.* Contrast-enhanced multidetector computed tomography viability imaging after myocardial infarction: characterization of myocyte death, microvascular obstruction, and chronic scar. Circulation 2006; 113(3): 394-404.
[http://dx.doi.org/10.1161/CIRCULATIONAHA.105.521450] [PMID: 16432071]

[204] Gerber BL, Belge B, Legros GJ, *et al.* Characterization of acute and chronic myocardial infarcts by multidetector computed tomography: comparison with contrast-enhanced magnetic resonance. Circulation 2006; 113(6): 823-33.
[http://dx.doi.org/10.1161/CIRCULATIONAHA.104.529511] [PMID: 16461822]

[205] Mahnken AH, Koos R, Katoh M, *et al.* Assessment of myocardial viability in reperfused acute myocardial infarction using 16-slice computed tomography in comparison to magnetic resonance imaging. J Am Coll Cardiol 2005; 45(12): 2042-7.
[http://dx.doi.org/10.1016/j.jacc.2005.03.035] [PMID: 15963407]

[206] Habis M, Capderou A, Ghostine S, *et al.* Acute myocardial infarction early viability assessment by 64-slice computed tomography immediately after coronary angiography: comparison with low-dose dobutamine echocardiography. J Am Coll Cardiol 2007; 49(11): 1178-85.
[http://dx.doi.org/10.1016/j.jacc.2006.12.032] [PMID: 17367662]

[207] Bauer RW, Kerl JM, Fischer N, *et al.* Dual-energy CT for the assessment of chronic myocardial infarction in patients with chronic coronary artery disease: comparison with 3-T MRI. AJR Am J Roentgenol 2010; 195(3): 639-46.
[http://dx.doi.org/10.2214/AJR.09.3849] [PMID: 20729440]

[208] Girsky MJ, Shinbane JS, Ahmadi N, Mao S, Flores F, Budoff MJ. Prospective randomized trial of venous cardiac computed tomographic angiography for facilitation of cardiac resynchronization therapy. Pacing Clin Electrophysiol 2010; 33(10): 1182-7.
[http://dx.doi.org/10.1111/j.1540-8159.2010.02821.x] [PMID: 20579305]

[209] Ortale JR, Gabriel EA, Iost C, Márquez CQ. The anatomy of the coronary sinus and its tributaries. Surg Radiol Anat 2001; 23(1): 15-21.
[http://dx.doi.org/10.1007/s00276-001-0015-0] [PMID: 11370136]

[210] Wang TJ, Larson MG, Levy D, *et al.* Temporal relations of atrial fibrillation and congestive heart failure and their joint influence on mortality: the Framingham Heart Study. Circulation 2003; 107(23): 2920-5.
[http://dx.doi.org/10.1161/01.CIR.0000072767.89944.6E] [PMID: 12771006]

[211] Masoudi FA, Calkins H, Kavinsky CJ, *et al.* 2015 ACC/HRS/SCAI Left Atrial Appendage Occlusion Device Societal Overview: A professional societal overview from the American College of Cardiology, Heart Rhythm Society, and Society for Cardiovascular Angiography and Interventions. Catheter Cardiovasc Interv 2015; 86(5): 791-807.
[http://dx.doi.org/10.1002/ccd.26170] [PMID: 26256562]

[212] Romero J, Husain SA, Kelesidis I, Sanz J, Medina HM, Garcia MJ. Detection of left atrial appendage thrombus by cardiac computed tomography in patients with atrial fibrillation: a meta-analysis. Circ Cardiovasc Imaging 2013; 6(2): 185-94.
[http://dx.doi.org/10.1161/CIRCIMAGING.112.000153] [PMID: 23406625]

[213] Lockwood SM, Alison JF, Obeyesekere MN, Mottram PM. Imaging the left atrial appendage prior to, during, and after occlusion. JACC Cardiovasc Imaging 2011; 4(3): 303-6.
[http://dx.doi.org/10.1016/j.jcmg.2010.09.024] [PMID: 21414580]

[214] Acharya D, Singh S, Tallaj JA, *et al.* Use of gated cardiac computed tomography angiography in the assessment of left ventricular assist device dysfunction. ASAIO J 2011; 57(1): 32-7.
[http://dx.doi.org/10.1097/MAT.0b013e3181fd3405] [PMID: 20966744]

[215] Raman SV, Sahu A, Merchant AZ, Louis LB IV, Firstenberg MS, Sun B. Noninvasive assessment of left ventricular assist devices with cardiovascular computed tomography and impact on management. J

Heart Lung Transplant 2010; 29(1): 79-85.
[http://dx.doi.org/10.1016/j.healun.2009.06.023] [PMID: 19782594]

[216] Scheske JA, O'Brien JM, Earls JP, *et al.* Coronary artery imaging with single-source rapid kilovolt peak-switching dual-energy CT. Radiology 2013; 268(3): 702-9.
[http://dx.doi.org/10.1148/radiol.13121901] [PMID: 23579045]

[217] Achenbach S, Marwan M, Schepis T, *et al.* High-pitch spiral acquisition: a new scan mode for coronary CT angiography. J Cardiovasc Comput Tomogr 2009; 3(2): 117-21.
[http://dx.doi.org/10.1016/j.jcct.2009.02.008] [PMID: 19332343]

[218] Lell M, Marwan M, Schepis T, *et al.* Prospectively ECG-triggered high-pitch spiral acquisition for coronary CT angiography using dual source CT: technique and initial experience. Eur Radiol 2009; 19(11): 2576-83.
[http://dx.doi.org/10.1007/s00330-009-1558-4] [PMID: 19760421]

[219] Schuleri KH, Centola M, Choi SH, *et al.* CT for evaluation of myocardial cell therapy in heart failure: a comparison with CMR imaging. JACC Cardiovasc Imaging 2011; 4(12): 1284-93.
[http://dx.doi.org/10.1016/j.jcmg.2011.09.013] [PMID: 22172785]

[220] Flotats A, Carrió I. Radionuclide noninvasive evaluation of heart failure beyond left ventricular function assessment. J Nucl Cardiol 2009; 16(2): 304-15.
[http://dx.doi.org/10.1007/s12350-009-9064-2] [PMID: 19247733]

[221] Carrió I. Cardiac neurotransmission imaging. J Nucl Med 2001; 42(7): 1062-76.
[PMID: 11438630]

[222] Bengel FM, Schwaiger M. Assessment of cardiac sympathetic neuronal function using PET imaging. J Nucl Cardiol 2004; 11(5): 603-16.
[http://dx.doi.org/10.1016/j.nuclcard.2004.06.133] [PMID: 15472645]

[223] Holly TA, Abbott BG, Al-Mallah M, *et al.* Single photon-emission computed tomography. J Nucl Cardiol 2010; 17(5): 941-73.
[http://dx.doi.org/10.1007/s12350-010-9246-y] [PMID: 20552312]

[224] Henzlova MJ, Cerqueira MD, Mahmarian JJ, Yao SS. Stress protocols and tracers. J Nucl Cardiol 2006; 13(6): e80-90.
[http://dx.doi.org/10.1016/j.nuclcard.2006.08.011] [PMID: 17174798]

[225] Abidov A, Hachamovitch R, Berman DS. Modern nuclear cardiac imaging in diagnosis and clinical management of patients with left ventricular dysfunction. Minerva Cardioangiol 2004; 52(6): 505-19.
[PMID: 15729211]

[226] Machac J, Bacharach SL, Bateman TM, *et al.* Positron emission tomography myocardial perfusion and glucose metabolism imaging. J Nucl Cardiol 2006; 13(6): e121-51.
[http://dx.doi.org/10.1016/j.nuclcard.2006.08.009] [PMID: 17174789]

[227] Duvall WL, Croft LB, Godiwala T, Ginsberg E, George T, Henzlova MJ. Reduced isotope dose with rapid SPECT MPI imaging: initial experience with a CZT SPECT camera. J Nucl Cardiol 2010; 17(6): 1009-14.
[http://dx.doi.org/10.1007/s12350-010-9215-5] [PMID: 21069489]

[228] Henzlova MJ, Duvall WL. The future of SPECT MPI: time and dose reduction. J Nucl Cardiol 2011; 18(4): 580-7.
[http://dx.doi.org/10.1007/s12350-011-9401-0] [PMID: 21638153]

[229] Maddox DE, Wynne J, Uren R, *et al.* Regional ejection fraction: a quantitative radionuclide index of regional left ventricular performance. Circulation 1979; 59(5): 1001-9.
[http://dx.doi.org/10.1161/01.CIR.59.5.1001] [PMID: 428081]

[230] Hesse B, Lindhardt TB, Acampa W, *et al.* EANM/ESC guidelines for radionuclide imaging of cardiac function. Eur J Nucl Med Mol Imaging 2008; 35(4): 851-85.
[http://dx.doi.org/10.1007/s00259-007-0694-9] [PMID: 18224320]

[231] Jessup M, Abraham WT, Casey DE, *et al.* 2009 focused update: ACCF/AHA Guidelines for the Diagnosis and Management of Heart Failure in Adults: a report of the American College of Cardiology Foundation/American Heart Association Task Force on Practice Guidelines: developed in collaboration with the International Society for Heart and Lung Transplantation. Circulation 2009; 119(14): 1977-2016.
[http://dx.doi.org/10.1161/CIRCULATIONAHA.109.192064] [PMID: 19324967]

[232] Mitra D, Basu S. Equilibrium radionuclide angiocardiography: Its usefulness in current practice and potential future applications. World J Radiol 2012; 4(10): 421-30.
[http://dx.doi.org/10.4329/wjr.v4.i10.421] [PMID: 23150766]

[233] Germano G, Kiat H, Kavanagh PB, *et al.* Automatic quantification of ejection fraction from gated myocardial perfusion SPECT. J Nucl Med 1995; 36(11): 2138-47.
[PMID: 7472611]

[234] Bavelaar-Croon CD, Pauwels EK, van der Wall EE. Gated single-photon emission computed tomographic myocardial imaging: a new tool in clinical cardiology. Am Heart J 2001; 141(3): 383-90.
[http://dx.doi.org/10.1067/mhj.2001.112780] [PMID: 11231435]

[235] Williams KA, Taillon LA. Left ventricular function in patients with coronary artery disease assessed by gated tomographic myocardial perfusion images. Comparison with assessment by contrast ventriculography and first-pass radionuclide angiography. J Am Coll Cardiol 1996; 27(1): 173-81.
[http://dx.doi.org/10.1016/0735-1097(95)00413-0] [PMID: 8522692]

[236] Ioannidis JP, Trikalinos TA, Danias PG. Electrocardiogram-gated single-photon emission computed tomography *versus* cardiac magnetic resonance imaging for the assessment of left ventricular volumes and ejection fraction: a meta-analysis. J Am Coll Cardiol 2002; 39(12): 2059-68.
[http://dx.doi.org/10.1016/S0735-1097(02)01882-X] [PMID: 12084609]

[237] Rajappan K, Livieratos L, Camici PG, Pennell DJ. Measurement of ventricular volumes and function: a comparison of gated PET and cardiovascular magnetic resonance. J Nucl Med 2002; 43(6): 806-10.
[PMID: 12050327]

[238] Sharir T, Germano G, Kang X, *et al.* Prediction of myocardial infarction *versus* cardiac death by gated myocardial perfusion SPECT: risk stratification by the amount of stress-induced ischemia and the poststress ejection fraction. J Nucl Med 2001; 42(6): 831-7.
[PMID: 11390544]

[239] Kim C, Kwok YS, Heagerty P, Redberg R. Pharmacologic stress testing for coronary disease diagnosis: A meta-analysis. Am Heart J 2001; 142(6): 934-44.
[http://dx.doi.org/10.1067/mhj.2001.119761] [PMID: 11717594]

[240] Nakata T, Hashimoto A, Wakabayashi T, Kusuoka H, Nishimura T. Prediction of new-onset refractory congestive heart failure using gated myocardial perfusion SPECT imaging in patients with known or suspected coronary artery disease subanalysis of the J-ACCESS database. JACC Cardiovasc Imaging 2009; 2(12): 1393-400.
[http://dx.doi.org/10.1016/j.jcmg.2009.09.010] [PMID: 20083074]

[241] Candell-Riera J, Romero-Farina G, Aguadé-Bruix S, Castell-Conesa J, de León G, García-Dorado D. Prognostic value of myocardial perfusion-gated SPECT in patients with ischemic cardiomyopathy. J Nucl Cardiol 2009; 16(2): 212-21.
[http://dx.doi.org/10.1007/s12350-008-9042-0] [PMID: 19159990]

[242] Mc Ardle BA, Dowsley TF, deKemp RA, Wells GA, Beanlands RS. Does rubidium-82 PET have superior accuracy to SPECT perfusion imaging for the diagnosis of obstructive coronary disease?: A systematic review and meta-analysis. J Am Coll Cardiol 2012; 60(18): 1828-37.
[http://dx.doi.org/10.1016/j.jacc.2012.07.038] [PMID: 23040573]

[243] Neglia D, Michelassi C, Trivieri MG, *et al.* Prognostic role of myocardial blood flow impairment in idiopathic left ventricular dysfunction. Circulation 2002; 105(2): 186-93.
[http://dx.doi.org/10.1161/hc0202.102119] [PMID: 11790699]

[244] Rijnierse MT, de Haan S, Harms HJ, *et al.* Impaired hyperemic myocardial blood flow is associated with inducibility of ventricular arrhythmia in ischemic cardiomyopathy. Circ Cardiovasc Imaging 2014; 7(1): 20-30.
[http://dx.doi.org/10.1161/CIRCIMAGING.113.001158] [PMID: 24343851]

[245] Tio RA, Dabeshlim A, Siebelink HM, *et al.* Comparison between the prognostic value of left ventricular function and myocardial perfusion reserve in patients with ischemic heart disease. J Nucl Med 2009; 50(2): 214-9.
[http://dx.doi.org/10.2967/jnumed.108.054395] [PMID: 19164219]

[246] Majmudar MD, Murthy VL, Shah RV, *et al.* Quantification of coronary flow reserve in patients with ischaemic and non-ischaemic cardiomyopathy and its association with clinical outcomes. Eur Heart J Cardiovasc Imaging 2015; 16(8): 900-9.
[http://dx.doi.org/10.1093/ehjci/jev012] [PMID: 25719181]

[247] Allman KC, Shaw LJ, Hachamovitch R, Udelson JE. Myocardial viability testing and impact of revascularization on prognosis in patients with coronary artery disease and left ventricular dysfunction: a meta-analysis. J Am Coll Cardiol 2002; 39(7): 1151-8.
[http://dx.doi.org/10.1016/S0735-1097(02)01726-6] [PMID: 11923039]

[248] Klocke FJ, Baird MG, Lorell BH, *et al.* ACC/AHA/ASNC guidelines for the clinical use of cardiac radionuclide imaging--executive summary: a report of the American College of Cardiology/American Heart Association Task Force on Practice Guidelines (ACC/AHA/ASNC Committee to Revise the 1995 Guidelines for the Clinical Use of Cardiac Radionuclide Imaging). J Am Coll Cardiol 2003; 42(7): 1318-33.
[http://dx.doi.org/10.1016/j.jacc.2003.08.011] [PMID: 14522503]

[249] Bax JJ, Wijns W, Cornel JH, Visser FC, Boersma E, Fioretti PM. Accuracy of currently available techniques for prediction of functional recovery after revascularization in patients with left ventricular dysfunction due to chronic coronary artery disease: comparison of pooled data. J Am Coll Cardiol 1997; 30(6): 1451-60.
[http://dx.doi.org/10.1016/S0735-1097(97)00352-5] [PMID: 9362401]

[250] Partington SL, Kwong RY, Dorbala S. Multimodality imaging in the assessment of myocardial viability. Heart Fail Rev 2011; 16(4): 381-95.
[http://dx.doi.org/10.1007/s10741-010-9201-7] [PMID: 21069458]

[251] Gibson RS, Watson DD, Taylor GJ, *et al.* Prospective assessment of regional myocardial perfusion before and after coronary revascularization surgery by quantitative thallium-201 scintigraphy. J Am Coll Cardiol 1983; 1(3): 804-15.
[http://dx.doi.org/10.1016/S0735-1097(83)80194-6] [PMID: 6600759]

[252] Schinkel AF, Bax JJ, Poldermans D, Elhendy A, Ferrari R, Rahimtoola SH. Hibernating myocardium: diagnosis and patient outcomes. Curr Probl Cardiol 2007; 32(7): 375-410.
[http://dx.doi.org/10.1016/j.cpcardiol.2007.04.001] [PMID: 17560992]

[253] Di Carli MF, Davidson M, Little R, *et al.* Value of metabolic imaging with positron emission tomography for evaluating prognosis in patients with coronary artery disease and left ventricular dysfunction. Am J Cardiol 1994; 73(8): 527-33.
[http://dx.doi.org/10.1016/0002-9149(94)90327-1] [PMID: 8147295]

[254] Nishiyama Y, Yamamoto Y, Fukunaga K, *et al.* Comparative evaluation of 18F-FDG PET and 67Ga scintigraphy in patients with sarcoidosis. J Nucl Med 2006; 47(10): 1571-6.
[PMID: 17015889]

[255] Youssef G, Leung E, Mylonas I, *et al.* The use of 18F-FDG PET in the diagnosis of cardiac sarcoidosis: a systematic review and metaanalysis including the Ontario experience. J Nucl Med 2012; 53(2): 241-8.
[http://dx.doi.org/10.2967/jnumed.111.090662] [PMID: 22228794]

[256] Betensky BP, Tschabrunn CM, Zado ES, *et al.* Long-term follow-up of patients with cardiac

sarcoidosis and implantable cardioverter-defibrillators. Heart Rhythm 2012; 9(6): 884-91.
[http://dx.doi.org/10.1016/j.hrthm.2012.02.010] [PMID: 22338670]

[257] Yamagishi H, Shirai N, Takagi M, *et al.* Identification of cardiac sarcoidosis with (13)N-NH(3)/(18)-
-FDG PET. J Nucl Med 2003; 44(7): 1030-6.
[PMID: 12843216]

[258] Ungerer M, Böhm M, Elce JS, Erdmann E, Lohse MJ. Altered expression of beta-adrenergic receptor
kinase and beta 1-adrenergic receptors in the failing human heart. Circulation 1993; 87(2): 454-63.
[http://dx.doi.org/10.1161/01.CIR.87.2.454] [PMID: 8381058]

[259] Nakata T, Wakabayashi T, Kyuma M, Takahashi T, Tsuchihashi K, Shimamoto K. Cardiac
metaiodobenzylguanidine activity can predict the long-term efficacy of angiotensin-converting
enzyme inhibitors and/or beta-adrenoceptor blockers in patients with heart failure. Eur J Nucl Med
Mol Imaging 2005; 32(2): 186-94.
[http://dx.doi.org/10.1007/s00259-004-1624-8] [PMID: 15452671]

[260] Barron HV, Lesh MD. Autonomic nervous system and sudden cardiac death. J Am Coll Cardiol 1996;
27(5): 1053-60.
[http://dx.doi.org/10.1016/0735-1097(95)00615-X] [PMID: 8609321]

[261] Somsen GA, Verberne HJ, Fleury E, Righetti A. Normal values and within-subject variability of
cardiac I-123 MIBG scintigraphy in healthy individuals: implications for clinical studies. J Nucl
Cardiol 2004; 11(2): 126-33.
[http://dx.doi.org/10.1016/j.nuclcard.2003.10.010] [PMID: 15052243]

[262] Jacobson AF, Senior R, Cerqueira MD, *et al.* Myocardial iodine-123 meta-iodobenzylguanidine
imaging and cardiac events in heart failure. Results of the prospective ADMIRE-HF (AdreView
Myocardial Imaging for Risk Evaluation in Heart Failure) study. J Am Coll Cardiol 2010; 55(20):
2212-21.
[http://dx.doi.org/10.1016/j.jacc.2010.01.014] [PMID: 20188504]

[263] Khaw BA, Fallon JT, Beller GA, Haber E. Specificity of localization of myosin-specific antibody
fragments in experimental myocardial infarction. Histologic, histochemical, autoradiographic and
scintigraphic studies. Circulation 1979; 60(7): 1527-31.
[http://dx.doi.org/10.1161/01.CIR.60.7.1527] [PMID: 498480]

[264] Narula J, Acio ER, Narula N, *et al.* Annexin-V imaging for noninvasive detection of cardiac allograft
rejection. Nat Med 2001; 7(12): 1347-52.
[http://dx.doi.org/10.1038/nm1201-1347] [PMID: 11726976]

CHAPTER 6

Cardiac Catheterization and Endomyocardial Biopsy for the Diagnosis of Heart Failure in Children

Ralf J. Holzer[1,*] and **Ziyad M. Hijazi[2]**

[1] *Weill Cornell Medicine, NewYork-Presbyterian Komansky Children's Hospital,USA*

[2] *Sidra Medicine, Doha-Qatar and Weill Cornell Medical Medicine, New York, USA*

Abstract: The most likely etiology of cardiac failure in neonates, children and young adults varies greatly by age and is often different from the type of etiology seen in adult patients. As such, the need for cardiac catheterization and endomyocardial biopsy depends on the (potential) underlying diagnosis and has to be carefully evaluated for every case, including the need for anesthesia, angiography and cardiac output evaluations.

Keywords: Cardiac Actheterization, Endomyocardial Biopsy, Pediatrics.

INTRODUCTION

Hemodynamic cardiac catheterizations combined with angiography and endomyocardial biopsy are some of the tools utilized in the diagnosis and management of congestive heart failure in children and young adults with congenital and acquired heart disease. While long being established diagnostic methods, there still appears to be confusion among practicing physicians as when to use these tools in the management of patients with heart failure. Furthermore there is not only confusion about the "when" but also a lack of understanding the "how" as it relates to obtaining and interpreting the hemodynamic data. Describing these evaluations purely as "just recording pressures" without much thought surrounding the procedure and the data that can be obtained would do injustice to the complexity of these evaluations and ignore the wide spectrum of data that can be gathered. This chapter describes in a brief and straightforward fashion the role and indication that cardiac catheterization and endomyocardial

---

* **Corresponding author Ralf J. Holzer:** Weill Cornell Medicine, Department of Pediatrics, 525 East 68th Street, New York, NY 10065, USA; Tel 212.746.3561; E-mail: rjh3001@med.cornell.edu

Mohammad El Tahlawi (Ed.)
All rights reserved-© 2020 Bentham Science Publishers

biopsy has in the management of children and young adults with congenital heart disease.

HEMODYNAMIC CARDIAC CATHETERIZATION

Indications

The indication and purpose of cardiac catheterization depend on several important factors, such as age, whether a specific underlying diagnosis is suspected or has been established, the need for a pre-transplant evaluation, or the assessment of the effects adjuvant drug therapy that is being delivered.

Age of clinical presentation alone is of great importance in pediatric patients, as many conditions present at fairly specific age ranges, and therefore become important differentials when evaluating these patients. For example, in a neonate and young infant with specific EKG changes and poor ventricular function, it will become an immediate necessity to delineate the origins of the coronary arteries to rule out an abnormal origin of a coronary artery, and if identified, to further delineate the origin of this vessel (such as for example from the pulmonary artery) (Figs. **1a-c**). In these patients, angiographic data obtained in the cardiac catheteri-

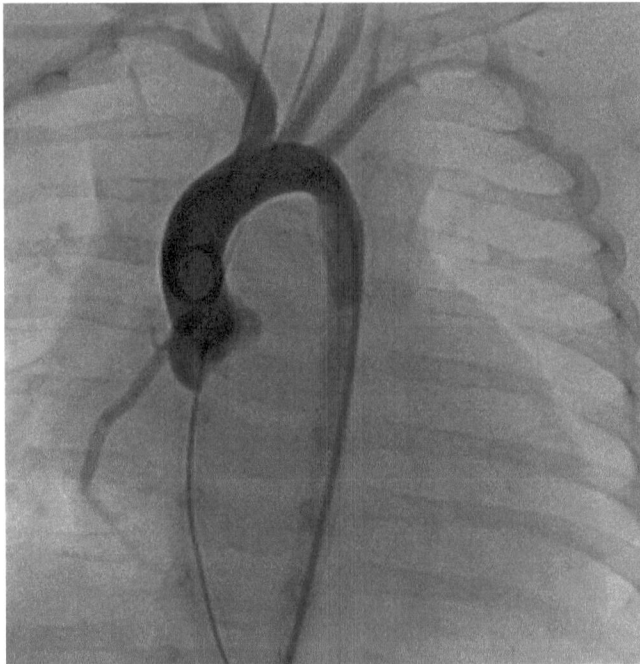

a

Fig. 1 cont.....

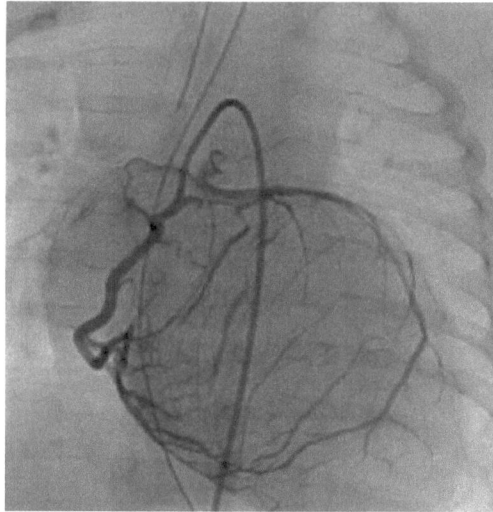

b

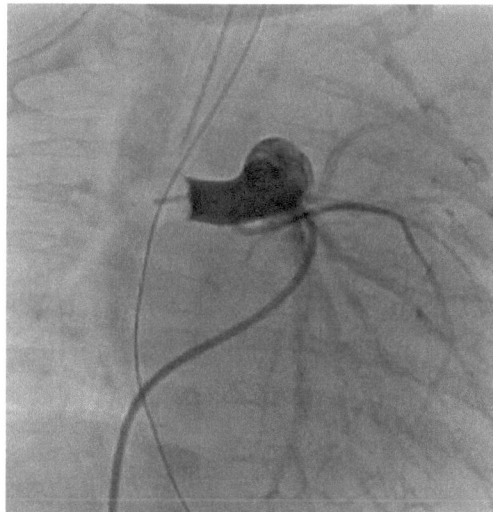

c

Fig. (1). Anomalous origin of the left coronary artery from the main pulmonary artery.
Two-month-old male infant presenting with symptoms and signs of cardiac failure and poor left ventricular function. Cardiac catheterization revealed a left ventricular end-diastolic pressure of 14mmHg. An angiography in the aorta (Fig. **1a**) documented only a right coronary artery. A selective injection in the right coronary artery demonstrated filling of the left coronary artery *via* collaterals and possible origin from the main pulmonary artery (Fig. **1b**). A final angiogram in the right pulmonary artery with occlusion of the distal vessel using a Berman angiographic catheter documented filling of the left coronary artery originating from RPA/MPA.

catheterization laboratory is most important, and hemodynamic data would be of secondary importance. The threshold to take a patient to the cath lab for evaluation of the coronary arteries is much lower in a neonate and young infant, as the above condition usually presents at a very young age when the pulmonary vascular resistance drops, thereby impacting the flow from main pulmonary artery into an abnormally originating coronary artery.

While the heightened concern about the presence of coronary artery abnormalities in neonates and young infants with impaired ventricular function is similar to adult patients, where often coronary artery disease is the main cause of unexplained congestive cardiac failure, this is in sharp contrast to many older pediatric patients beyond infancy, who usually have neither congenital nor acquired coronary artery disease, and where the main purpose of cardiac catheterization in patients with congestive cardiac failure often is either a pre-transplant evaluation of pulmonary artery pressures and vascular resistance, a hemodynamic evaluation at the same time as obtaining an endomyocardial biopsy, or a complex functional assessment as part of an overall management plan of patients with chronic congestive cardiac failure. This does also include the evaluation of drug therapies, such as inotropes or vasodilators, where data obtained prior to and after a period of therapy may provide useful data to assess the response to therapy.

Older patients with chronic congestive cardiac failure on the background of palliated congenital heart disease are another group of patients, where there often is a need for not just a hemodynamic evaluation, but where the procedure is performed to frequently deliver transcatheter therapies to palliate or treat potential anatomic and/or structural problems at the same time.

What is most important in evaluating any of these patients, is to have a well-defined plan on what data would need to be obtained in the catheterization laboratory, and how this data would integrate into the management plan of the patient, irrespective of whether this is angiographic or hemodynamic data. One should critically question the value of any invasive procedure that is being performed in any patient and assess whether the needed data can be obtained using other less invasive modalities. It is important to clearly state what exact hemodynamic data will need to be obtained and critically evaluate whether the result may lead to a change in the management of the patient (*e.g.* does it make a difference, whether the LVEDP is identified to be 21 instead of 13 – would that change the management of the patient?), or whether it provides important prognostic data. If the results will not change the management, is the procedure really needed? Are there alternative methods to obtaining the required data (such as a CT or MRI)? Given that every diagnostic cardiac catheterization is an invasive procedure with a small risk, especially in patients with compromised ventricular function, an approach that utilizes cardiac catheterization to "just obtain the pressures" without a thoughtful plan on why this data is important, is not adequate and exposes the patient to unnecessary risks.

Procedural Considerations, Technique, and Hemodynamic Evaluation

Evaluating a patient with congestive cardiac failure in the catheterization laboratory has to be planned very carefully in conjunction with a dedicated pediatric cardiac anesthetist. Many agents used for induction and maintenance of anesthesia can have an effect on systemic and pulmonary vascular resistance, and may drop the blood pressure to varying degrees. Performing a procedure using local anesthesia often provides better hemodynamic stability, but in young children this is rarely feasible without additional sedation. If transcatheter interventions are planned or considered during the procedure, then general anesthesia may be more appropriate and allows better control during the procedure, but the operator will need to be aware and conscious of the effects of anesthetic agents on the obtained hemodynamic data. Equally, in patients with single ventricle physiology and congestive cardiac failure, positive pressure ventilation may have a negative impact on the pressures that are recorded within a Glenn or Fontan circulation. Irrespective of whether the procedure is performed under general anesthesia or with just a sedating agent, it is important to have the case monitored by a dedicated pediatric cardiac anesthetist to provide the greatest procedural safety net, as the hemodynamic status in these patients can deteriorate quickly, requiring the full focus and attention of the physician monitoring the patient.

A decision has to be made as to whether just an isolated right heart catheterization is required, or whether additionally a retrograde left heart catheterization should be performed. By and large, in most patients, a right heart catheterization with pulmonary capillary wedge pressures in combination with arterial monitoring of the systemic blood pressure is adequate. This setup allows obtaining of arterial blood gasses, calculation of pulmonary and systemic vascular resistances, and provides a crucial safety net by being able to monitor these fragile patients adequately during the procedure. If an aortogram or ventriculogram are necessary, or if there are concerns of other structural problems that may require measurement of left ventricular pressures (such as concerns of mitral valve or pulmonary vein stenosis), then a full retrograde left heart cardiac catheterization should be performed, unless of course a patent foramen ovale or atrial septal defect is present, which would allow a left heart catheterization to be performed antegradely through the atrial communication. However, if a retrograde catheterization is required, care has to be taken in patients where there is a suspicion of coronary abnormalities, as retrograde crossing the aortic valve with a somewhat stiff pigtail catheter, may temporarily reduce the coronary perfusion pressure and can lead to significant hemodynamic instability or arrhythmias. This is particular important in infants, where a 4Fr pigtail catheter can easily splint one of the cusps of the aortic valve. In those scenarios, sometimes crossing the aortic valve with a soft 0.014" pressure wire may alleviate that concern, while still allowing obtaining all the required hemodynamic data. Alternatively, even though we would usually recommend performing angiographies only after completing the hemodynamic evaluation, in patients with suspected coronary artery anomalies, an initial screening aortogram may be helpful prior to completing the rest of the hemodynamic evaluation.

All planning related to the procedure, anesthesia, and required data should be performed well in advance and not at the day of cardiac catheterization. Once the patient is sedated or anesthetized and/or local anesthesia has been administered, vascular access is obtained and usually small sheath sizes are sufficient to accommodate the catheters required for a standalone hemodynamic evaluation. Patients with congestive cardiac failure are at increased risk of thrombus formation, so Heparin should be administered and monitored with the activated clotting time. Exceptions are patients that require endomyocardial biopsy where the administration of Heparin is usually delayed until the biopsy has been performed. A standard right heart catheterization is performed once the patient is hemodynamically stable and ideally maintained in room air. Patients that are critically ill and who are maintained on oxygen and/or inotropic support prior to arriving at the catheterization laboratory should be maintained on the same amount of oxygen and inotropes in the cath lab that they were maintained on while in the critical care unit. Any attempts at weaning oxygen or vasoactive substances should be completed at least 24 hours prior to the procedure, to avoid a situation where the data obtained in the catheterization laboratory reflects the withdrawal of these medications, potentially leading to a deterioration of the clinical status at the time of cardiac catheterization.

All data obtained in the catheterization laboratory needs to be carefully reviewed and interpreted during the procedure, and if/when needed, repeated as to have accurate data to base clinical decisions upon. If there is a concern about pulmonary vascular resistance, data will need to be repeated with 100% oxygen +/- Nitric Oxide at 80 ppm. It is important that sufficient time is allowed to reach a steady state (usually about 10 minutes) and then the evaluation performed quickly, prior to reducing/eliminating oxygen and pulmonary vasodilators to baseline settings. Remaining on high doses of pulmonary vasodilators for too long, risks potential re-bound pulmonary hypertension, in particular in patients with baseline elevated pulmonary vascular resistance.

The cardiac output can be estimated using the Fick principle, with oxygen consumption being estimated using either the LaFarge method for patients above 3 years of age, or the modified formula by Lundell and colleagues for patients below the age of 3 years [1]. Any interpretation of clinical data has to be carefully reviewed within the clinical context of the patient, and it is important to be aware of the many assumptions that are made to allow using the Fick principle with oxygen consumption. An alternative method for evaluating the cardiac output is thermodilution. However, the required catheters are not always very accurate and results not always reproducible, in particular in pediatric patients. We have found a wide variety of results obtained in pediatric patients, which is particularly important in patients with low cardiac output where thermodilution tends to overestimate the cardiac output. We therefore do not advocate the use of thermodilution catheters on a regular basis in pediatric patients, or patients with congestive cardiac failure. Load independent parameters can be obtained using cardiac conductance catheters, but these are expensive, the setup is cumbersome, and in most centers this is used mainly as a research tool, rather than on a routine basis.

Important data elements to obtain and measure in any patient with congestive cardiac failure include the (left and right) ventricular end-diastolic pressures or at least the pulmonary capillary wedge pressures, the pulmonary artery pressures, as well as the pulmonary and systemic vascular resistance indexes. It is essential that any operator who performs these types of catheterizations is familiar with pressure curves and tracings, signs of restrictive cardiomyopathy *versus* pericarditis, as well as hemodynamic signs of hypertrophic cardiomyopathy (and how to evaluate it in the catheterization laboratory). If needed, intraoperative transesophageal or intracardiac echocardiography can be performed while under general anesthesia to correlate hemodynamic findings with echocardiographic appearance (such as large V-waves and mitral regurgitation).

Where needed, inotropic or fluid challenges should be performed. Evaluating the response to Dobutamine may aid in deciding whether this therapy may be beneficial to a specific patient. This is particularly important in patients who are close to be considered transplant candidates, where this therapy may be entertained for a prolonged period of time. For this purpose, once a basic set of hemodynamic data has been obtained, Dobutamine is commenced at doses between 5-10mcg/kg/min, usually starting at the lower end around 5 or 7.5mcg/kg/min. This should be administered through a central line or central vascular access where feasible and sufficient time should be allowed to clear the dead space and for the drug to reach the patient. One of the biggest mistakes in prematurely increasing the dose of Dobutamine without giving it sufficient time to take action, and then suddenly ending up with an unwanted excessively hypertensive response, which can be detrimental in these patient. Again, it may take some time before a steady state has been reached, depending on the volume that has to be cleared through the line and having an appropriate carrier fluid rate is important in this context.

Volume challenges are less frequently needed in the evaluations of patients with congestive cardiac failure. It may be useful in patients where hemodynamic data look surprisingly "normal", but where an extra fluid administration may lead to an increase in end-diastolic pressures due to the shift on the starling curve to the right (beyond its peak), combined with a drop in cardiac output. However, this is rarely needed as the documentation of congestive cardiac failure using a combination of clinical signs, symptoms and echocardiography is usually adequate with very little benefit of artificially increasing the enddiastolic pressure through fluid administration. If fluid is administered, it should be usually at a dose of 10-20ml /kg of normal saline administered fairly rapidly (but while carefully monitoring the pressures), with hemodynamic data being obtained immediately thereafter. The effect usually wears off fairly quickly, and therefore waiting is unwanted in this scenario.

Once all hemodynamic data has been obtained and reviewed, then if needed this is followed by endomyocardial biopsy and any transcatheter intervention that may be required in the patient.

ENDOMYOCARDIAL BIOPSY

Indications

In pediatric patients, the most common primary causes of congestive cardiac failure include underlying congenital heart disease, idiopathic dilated cardiomyopathy and viral myocarditis, as well as some hereditary metabolic disorders. When considering an endomyocardial biopsy in a pediatric patient with congestive cardiac failure, it is important to not just consider the value and yield of endomyocardial biopsy in isolation, but to evaluate it on the background of the suspected diagnosis, the procedural risks, the potential therapeutic implications, as well as the availability of other less invasive diagnostic methods such as cardiac MRI, viral testing, as well as metabolic and genetic screening. Cardiac MRI in particular has an excellent sensitivity in diagnosing acute myocarditis (*versus* chronic myocarditis), even though it does not help identifying a possible viral etiology [2].

In general, data relating to the usefulness of endomyocardial biopsy specific to pediatric patients with cardiomyopathy is scarce. As far back as 1988, Leather-bury and colleagues reported a change in diagnosis in 8 out of 16 patients with dilated cardiomyopathy as a result of obtaining an endomyocardial biopsy, which included myocarditis, carnitine deficiency, and hypertrophic cardiomyopathy, all conditions that in the modern area can be diagnosed using a combination of cardiovascular MRI and genetic/ metabolic testing [3].

A scientific statement by the American Heart Association and the American College of Cardiology (adult and pediatric patients) suggested an important diagnostic benefit in the evaluation of patients with non-ischemic congestive cardiac failure [4]. The statement listed indications that were based on comparing the potential yield and benefit in terms of diagnostic, prognostic, and therapeutic decision making with the procedural risks of adverse events. Specifically, class I indications for endomyocardial biopsy for both, adult and pediatric patients, included new-onset heart failure of less than 2 weeks duration with hemodynamic compromise (irrespective of presence of a dilated LV), and new onset heart failure of 2 weeks to 3 month duration with a dilated ventricle and either ventricular arrhythmias, or second or third degree heart block, or failure to respond to usual care within 1-2 weeks (if duration > 3months, then this would fall under class IIa). Additional class IIa indications include heart failure associated with anthracycline chemotherapy or an unexplained restrictive cardiomyopathy, suspected cardiac tumors, unexplained cardiomyopathy in children, or heart failure associated with dilated cardiomyopathy associated with suspected allergic reaction or eosinophilia [4].

It is important to always evaluate the potential benefit of endomyocardial biopsy in the context of possible procedure related adverse events. The most current data on the safety and diagnostic yield of endomyocardial biopsy in pediatric heart transplant recipients was reported from the C3PO registry, with a 3.3% overall rate of adverse events, and 1.1% rate of high severity adverse events, with 19% of adverse events being classified as biopsy-related, including tricuspid valve injury and complete heart block [5]. Myocardial perforation was not observed in any case. Only about 1% of cases had non-diagnostic specimens obtained. While not specifically evaluated in that study, risks are likely higher in very small patients with additional data originating from the C3PO registry having found a weight of less than 2kg as an additional independent risk factor for adverse events [6].

Interestingly, the C3PO data also documented that adverse events related to coronary angiography (if combined with endomyocardial biopsy) were observed in 1.2% of cases, and this data suggested that even though the risks of endomyocardial biopsy are very low, combining endomyocardial biopsy with coronary angiography tripled the risk of adverse events during the procedure, and therefore careful consideration should be given as to whether selective coronary angiography is required.

Unfortunately, the AHA and ACC guidelines have not been revised recently and for the pediatric population, the therapeutic implications are limited in pediatric patients with unexplained heart failure, with frequently no significant difference in the (supportive) treatment that is being offered irrespective of the diagnostic results of the biopsy (which usually also includes administration of intravenous immunoglobulin as well as carnitine supplementation). While biopsy may give useful prognostic information, it is presently less commonly performed in pediatric patients with newly diagnosed congestive cardiac failure, even those with acute presentation. However, decisions need to be made on a case-by-case basis of whether to consider endomyocardial biopsy or not.

Procedural and Technical Considerations

Given that endomyocardial biopsy is usually combined with hemodynamic cardiac catheterization, general pre-procedural considerations are the same as those for an isolated hemodynamic cardiac catheterization. The biopsy is usually deferred until after the hemodynamic evaluation is completed, to avoid those arrhythmias and conduction abnormalities may render the obtained hemodynamic data useless. Heparin is only administered after the biopsy is obtained, provided additional angiographies or interventions need to be performed, in particular in patients where an arterial sheath has been placed.

The technique of endomyocardial biopsy has been described in many textbooks and articles, so we only briefly highlight some of the important consideration. Standard right ventricular biopsy can be performed using an internal jugular venous or a femoral venous approach. If no retrograde arterial catheterization is required, the internal jugular venous approach is usually preferable, while the femoral venous approach is more practical when also performing retrograde left ventricular catheterization or coronary angiography. Imamura and colleagues reported significantly shorter procedure times and radiation dose when using the internal jugular venous *versus* the femoral venous approach in adult patients [7].

The size of the bioptome and selection of the long sheath should be adjusted according to patient size and the approach that has been chosen. In general it is preferable to not cross the tricuspid valve directly with the bioptome, as this can lead to tricuspid valve injury. It is recommended to position the chosen long sheath within the right atrium, and then advance a balloon wedge catheter into the right atrium, inflate the balloon, and across the tricuspid valve into the right ventricle. This then allows advancing the long sheath over the wedge catheter and towards the right ventricular apex. Care has to be taken to diligently aspirate and flush the sheath to avoid any inadvertent air embolism (and repeat this each time a specimen has been obtained). It has been our practice to use sheaths with side-holes, if not available, we make some side-holes near the tip of the sheath. The presence of these side-holes allows easier aspiration and flushing without the fear of air introduction into the system. It is also helpful to pre-curve the bioptome (with the forceps opened) as to allow directing it more posteriorly towards the interventricular septum. A straight left anterior oblique projection is usually best to profile the ventricular septum (combined with lateral projection), and the bioptome is advanced to the tip of the sheath, the sheath is retracted over the bioptome, and then the bioptome is opened, advanced forward towards the septum, then closed and retracted into the sheath. This process is repeated until about 5 specimens are obtained, repositioning the sheath at least once in the process. The obtained specimens should be evaluated briefly by a member of the pathology team to affirm, that they are sufficient for the tests that are being considered.

While right ventricular endomyocardial biopsy is most frequently performed in pediatric patients, left ventricular biopsy can be considered as an alternative technique in larger patients. Adult studies have shown no significant differences in diagnostic results and procedure related major adverse events when comparing right ventricular to left ventricular biopsy [8]. Contraindications to left ventricular endomyocardial biopsy include left ventricular non-compaction or aortic valve stenosis. Specific techniques such as performing left ventricular biopsy using transradial access and a guide catheter have been described in adults, but are not feasible options in pediatric patients [9]. At the end of the biopsy, repeat hemodynamic assessment is performed to monitor the right ventricular enddiastolic pressure. Also, a transthoracic echocardiogram is obtained to rule out presence of any pericardial effusion.

SUMMARY

As a summary, this chapter outlines some of the important considerations when evaluating pediatric patients with congestive cardiac failure in the catheterization laboratory. Pre-procedural planning is crucial and a diligent review of the recorded data is required at the time of the procedure. The use of endomyocardial biopsy in pediatric patients with congestive cardiac failure should be considered in selected patients.

CONSENT FOR PUBLICATION

Not applicable.

CONFLICT OF INTEREST

The authors confirm that this chapter contents have no conflict of interest.

ACKNOWLEDGEMENTS

Declared none.

REFERENCES

[1]   Lundell BP, Casas ML, Wallgren CG. Oxygen consumption in infants and children during heart catheterization. Pediatr Cardiol 1996; 17(4): 207-13.
[http://dx.doi.org/10.1007/BF02524795] [PMID: 8662051]

[2]   Lurz P, Eitel I, Adam J, *et al.* Diagnostic performance of CMR imaging compared with EMB in patients with suspected myocarditis. JACC Cardiovasc Imaging 2012; 5(5): 513-24.
[http://dx.doi.org/10.1016/j.jcmg.2011.11.022] [PMID: 22595159]

[3]   Leatherbury L, Chandra RS, Shapiro SR, Perry LW. Value of endomyocardial biopsy in infants, children and adolescents with dilated or hypertrophic cardiomyopathy and myocarditis. J Am Coll Cardiol 1988; 12(6): 1547-54.
[http://dx.doi.org/10.1016/S0735-1097(88)80024-X] [PMID: 3192852]

[4]   Cooper LT, Baughman KL, Feldman AM, *et al.* The role of endomyocardial biopsy in the management of cardiovascular disease: A scientific statement from the American Heart Association, the American College of Cardiology, and the European Society of Cardiology. Circulation 2007; 116(19): 2216-33.
[http://dx.doi.org/10.1161/CIRCULATIONAHA.107.186093] [PMID: 17959655]

[5]   Daly KP, Marshall AC, Vincent JA, Zuckerman WA, Hoffman TM, Canter CE, *et al.* Endomyocardial biopsy and selective coronary angiography are low-risk procedures in pediatric heart transplant recipients: results of a multicenter experience The Journal of heart and lung transplantation : The official publication of the International Society for Heart Transplantation 2012; 31(4): 398-409.
[http://dx.doi.org/10.1016/j.healun.2011.11.019]

[6]   Backes CH, Cua C, Kreutzer J, Armsby L, El-Said H, Moore JW, *et al.* Low weight as an independent risk factor for adverse events during cardiac catheterization of infants Catheterization and cardiovascular interventions : Official journal of the Society for Cardiac Angiography & Interventions 2013; 8(5): 786-94.
[http://dx.doi.org/10.1002/ccd.24726]

[7]   Imamura T, Kinugawa K, Nitta D, *et al.* Is the internal jugular vein or femoral vein a better approach site for endomyocardial biopsy in heart transplant recipients? Int Heart J 2015; 56(1): 67-72.
[http://dx.doi.org/10.1536/ihj.14-156] [PMID: 25503653]

[8]   Yilmaz A, Kindermann I, Kindermann M, *et al.* Comparative evaluation of left and right ventricular endomyocardial biopsy: differences in complication rate and diagnostic performance. Circulation 2010; 122(9): 900-9.
[http://dx.doi.org/10.1161/CIRCULATIONAHA.109.924167] [PMID: 20713901]

[9]   Schulz E, Jabs A, Gori T, Hink U, Sotiriou E, Tschope C, *et al.* Feasibility and safety of left ventricular endomyocardial biopsy *via* transradial access: Technique and initial experience Catheterization and cardiovascular interventions : Official journal of the Society for Cardiac Angiography & Interventions 2015.

CHAPTER 7

Surgical Treatment of Heart Failure

Anas Taqatqa[1], Mohammad El Tahlawi[2], Sawsan Awad[1,*] and Khaled Abdelhady[1]

[1] *Rush University Medical Center, Chicago, USA*

[2] *Zagazig University, Zagazig, Egypt*

Abstract: There are different interventional & surgical modalities for management of resistant or end-stage heart failure. Biventricular pacing and cardiac resynchronization therapy are used in patients with failed medical treatment. Implantable defibrillator could be implanted in patients with recorded syncope, aborted sudden death or malignant ventricular arrythmia. Mechanical circulatory support has been utilized as a bridge either to recovery in cases of reversible etiologies or heart transplantation in cases of irreversible causes.

Keywords: Biventricular Pacing, Cardiac Resynchronization Therapy, Congenital Heart Disease, End-Stage Heart Failure, Extracorporeal Membrane Oxygenation, Heart Transplantation, Implantable Cardioverter Defibrillator, Mechanical Circulatory Support, Surgical Treatment, Ventricular Assist Device.

BIVENTRICULAR PACING (CARDIAC RESYNCHRONIZATION THERAPY)

Cardiac resynchronization therapy (CRT) has been attempted successfully in adult patients with heart failure and ventricular dys-synchrony. CRT is a treatment modality for those patients with failed medical management in the form of persistent symptom and signs of HF. Candidates for CRT include symptomatic patients with NYHA class III/IV, patients with LV ejection fraction (EF) of less than 35% and wide QRS of more than 120 milliseconds. CRT improved HF symptoms in the above-mentioned categories. It also improved their quality of life documented by better exercise tolerance. CRT also impacted echocardiographic findings of HF with much improved parameters and finally, it reduced the mortality rate of patients with HF and failed medical therapy [1 - 3].

CRT indications in adult population cannot be applied to children. HF etiology in

* **Corresponding author Sawsan Awad:** Rush University Medical Center Chicago, IL 60612, USA; Tel: 1-216-7-2-8035; Email: sawsan _m _ awad @r ush. edu

Mohammad El Tahlawi (Ed.)
All rights reserved-© 2020 Bentham Science Publishers

pediatric age group is seldom similar to that in adult population. Patients with congenital heart disease (CHD), especially post-surgical repair, frequently require CRT [4].

Patients with systemic LV HF, as patients with normal cardiac anatomy and atrioventricular block or cardiomyopathy, respond well to CRT [5 - 7]. Parameters of improvement include decrease in LV dimension and increase in EF [8].

Systemic RV HF is commonly seen in patients with transposition of the great arteries (D-TGA) post Mustard and Senning procedures and in patients with congenitally corrected TGA (CC-TGA). Several reports showed improvement in symptoms, exercise performance and RV EF [9 - 11].

On the other hand, patients with CHD in the form of SV benefited from CRT to some extent. CRT led to improvement in blood pressure, cardiac indices, mechanical synchrony noted on echocardiography and improvement of the SV EF in several patients [6, 12, 13].

Mid and long-term outcomes following CRT in congenital heart disease patients have been investigated in several studies which showed improvement in the EF of the systemic ventricle and improvement of overall patients' survival [5 - 7]. Transvenous lead placement is a challenge in pediatric patients that is why surgical epicardial leads are placed more often than transvenous ones particularly in low weight patients or conjointly in patients needing surgical repair for their underlying CHD [4].

PACEMAKER AND IMPLANTABLE DEFIBRILLATOR THERAPY

Recommendations for pacemaker and defibrillator placement were reviewed by the AHA/ACC/HRS in 2008. It includes guidelines for placement in children with HF and CHD based on expert opinions. Pacemaker implantation is indicated in children with CHD and HF in cases of symptomatic bradycardia, AV dys-synchrony, or intra-atrial re-entrant tachyarrhythmias [14]. Implantable cardiac defibrillators are commonly used for secondary prevention in children with CHD who had one of the following conditions: aborted sudden cardiac death, syncopal episode or documented tachycardia following repair of TOF, D-TGA post Mustard or Senning procedure, post Fontan procedure and left heart obstructive lesions [15, 16]. In a recent study in patients awaiting heart transplantation, the overall incidence of sudden death was 1.3%, which discourages the use of universal placement of ICDs for primary prevention [14, 15, 17].

MECHANICAL CIRCULATORY SUPPORT AND HEART TRANSPLANTATION

HF in children might progress to advanced stages, even with optimal medical treatment; therefore heart transplantation (HT) becomes a therapeutic option. Nevertheless, HT is limited by the availability of suitable donor and viable hearts. The mortality rate in infants listed for a HT in USA reaches up to 25% [18] and in children up to 17% [19]. Mechanical circulatory support has been utilized as a bridge either to recovery in cases of reversible etiologies or heart transplantation in cases of irreversible causes. International Society for Heart and Lung Transplantation (ISHLT) reported that one quarter of children received HT was bridged by mechanical circulatory support [20].

Ventricular Assist Device (VAD)

Several types of VADs are currently available which vary in flow design, delivery system and pump location [21]. Berlin Excor VAD is a paracorporeal pulsatile device which offers either univentricular or biventricular support [22]. The FDA approved this device following a study comparing Berlin heart VAD to ECMO, which clearly indicated its longer-term benefit to support small children awaiting heart transplantation. Potential complications in patients supported on the Berlin heart VAD include gastrointestinal or intracranial bleeding, stroke and device related infections. It has been used successfully in small number of patients with SV, though its ability is inferior compared to biventricular patients. The outcome was superior in patients with Glenn or Fontan compared with patients following Sano or Blalock Tassing shunt [23].

Available VADs are either temporary or durable. Table **1** presents lists of some approved durable and temporary devices.

Table 1. Approved temporary and durable devices eligible for entry into pediMACS [24].

PediMACS Devices	
Durable	Temporary
AbioCor TAH,Abiomed, Inc.	Abiomed AB5000, Abiomed, Inc.
MicroMed Debakey VAD-Child, Micromed Technology, Inc	Abiomed BVS 5000, Abiomed, Inc.
SynCardia, Syncardia Systems, Inc.	Impella 2.5, Abiomed, Inc.
HeartMate II LVAS, Thoratec Corporation	Impella 5.0, Abiomed, Inc.
HeartMate IP, Thoratec Corporation	Impella CF, Abiomed, Inc.
HeartMate VE,Thoratec Corporation	Tandem Heart, CardiacAssist, Inc

(Table 1) cont.....

PediMACS Devices	
HeartMate XVE, Thoratec Corporation	Thoratec CentriMag, Thoratec Corporation, Inc
Thoratec IVAD, Thoratec Corporation	Thoratec PediMag, Thoratec Corporation, Inc.
Thoratec PVAD, Thoratec Corporation	Biomedicus, Medtronic Biomedicus, Inc.
HeartWare HVAD, HeartWare, Inc.	Jostra Rotaflow, Maquet Cardiovasuclar
NovaCor PC, HeartWare, Inc. NovaCor PCq, HeartWare, Inc. Berlin Heart EXCOR Pediatric, Berlin Heart, Inc.	Revolution, Sorin Group

Pediatric Interagency Registry for Mechanically Assisted Circulatory Support (PediMACS) was a prospective registry with pediatric enrollment of children and adolescents. It began in 2012 and now has 4200 patients enrolled from more than 37 centers [24].

Significant patient-device size mismatch increased with smaller hearts. The smaller the heart, the more significant the size mismatch between the patient and the device. Although initial reports with continuous-flow VADs in children are rather encouraging, it is premature to state that continuous-flow devices would have a good impact across the spectrum of body sizes in the pediatric population [25]. According to the first PediMACS registry, approximately 54% of the approved durable devices are continuous-flow devices [24]. The emergence of the Infant Jarvik 2015, the first continuous-flow device specifically designed for small children, may further increase the attitude toward the use of continuous-flow devices in pediatric populations [25].

In Nassar *et al* 2017 study [26], they found comparable outcomes between children and adolescents <16 years receiving implantable continuous flow VADs and a matched group of those receiving the well-established pulsatile flow paracorporeal LVAD Berlin Heart EXCOR® in terms of incidence of complications and overall event-free survival at 1 year.

The main advantage of continuous-flow VADs, is their portability, which allows easy discharge and early regaining of daily life activities [27]. This is a point that may improve the quality of life for those hospital-bound kids [26].

Extracorporeal Membrane Oxygenation (ECMO)

ECMO provides total cardiopulmonary support for children as a bridge to heart transplantation. Additional indications following cardiac surgery include: deteriorating low cardiac output syndrome and failure to disconnect from cardiopulmonary bypass circuit. Moreover, it has been a part of the cardiopulmonary resuscitation (E-CPR) protocol in some institutions [28]. It is used as a short-term bridge (days to weeks) to recovery, VAD or HT. Potential complications include bleeding (intracranial, cannula or surgical site), neurological (like strokes and seizures), circuit problems (like pump malfunction or oxygenator failure). The overall survival for cardiac ECMO according to the Extracorporeal Life Support Organization Registry (ELSO) is 40% in neonates and 49% in pediatric less than 16 year of age [29].

Complications of ECMO could be mechanical related to the device itself, hemostatic, infectious or organ damage.

Table **2** summarizes the adverse effects of ECMO.

Table 2. Adverse effects that could occur in pediatric patients with ECMO [30 - 33].

Mechanical Complications	Air entrainment and air embolism	Especially in neonates
	Displaced and malpositioned cannulae	may interrupt flow during ECMO
	Malfunction of the mechanical pump	
	Tube disconnection or rupture	
Hemostatic complications	Thrombosis and clot formation	coagulation and fibrinolytic pathway activation and a complement-mediated inflammatory response.
	Hemorrhagic complications	caused by excessive anticoagulation
	Thrombocytopenia	Heparin-induced thrombocytopenia (HIT) should be considered
	Hemodilution	
Infectious Complications	bloodstream infections, mediastinitis, cannula infections, and ventilator-associated pneumonia, severe sepsis or septic shock.	Increasing age of child is a risk factor
CNS & Other organ damage (Ischemic Complications)	Neurologic: cerebrovascular hemorrhage, ischemia, infarction	a major cause of death in the infant population
	Limb ischemia	Due to cannulation of the femoral artery in pediatric populations
	Acute kidney injury	
	Gastrointestinal bleed with perforation and ulceration	
	Hepatic failure	

The mortality of children requiring prolonged cardiac ECMO increases with prolonged duration (≥14 days), smaller weight and underlying congenital heart disease [34].

Heart Transplantation (HT)

More than ten thousand pediatric HT has been reported to the registry of ISHLT so far [35]. The American Heart Association published recommendations [36] for the indications for the pediatric heart transplant (Table **3**).

Table 3. Indications for pediatric HT.

Indications	Level of Evidence
Class I	
Stage D HF associated with systemic ventricular dysfunction in pediatric patients with cardiomyopathies or previously repaired/palliated CHD	B
Stage C HF associated with severe limitation of exercise and activity (peak maximum oxygen consumption <50% predicted for age and sex)	C
Stage C HF associated with systemic ventricular dysfunction in patients with cardiomyopathies or previously repaired/palliated CHD when HF is associated with significant growth failure attributable to the heart disease	B
Stage C HF associated near sudden death or life-threatening arrhythmias untreatable with medications or an ICD	C
Stage C HF in pediatric restrictive cardiomyopathy disease associated with reactive pulmonary hypertension	C
Class IIA	
Stage C HF in pediatric heart disease associated with reactive pulmonary hypertension and a potential risk of developing fixed, irreversible increase in pulmonary vascular resistance.	C
Anatomic and physiological conditions likely to worsen the natural history of CHD in infant patients with a single ventricle physiology, including: (1) severe stenosis or atresia in proximal coronary arteries; (2) moderate to severe stenosis or insufficiency of the AV or systemic semilunar valve(s); and (3) severe ventricular dysfunction.	C
Anatomic and physiological conditions likely to worsen the natural history of previously repaired or palliated CHD in patients with stage C heart failure without severe systemic ventricular dysfunction, including (1) pulmonary hypertension at risk of developing fixed, irreversible increase in pulmonary vascular resistance (2) severe aortic or systemic atrioventricular valve insufficiency that is not considered amenable to surgical correction; (3) severe arterial oxygen desaturation (cyanosis) not amenable to surgical correction; and (4) persistent protein-losing enteropathy despite optimal medical/surgical therapy.	C
HF: heart failure. ICD: implantable cardioverter defibrillator. CHD: congenital heart disease. Stage A HF: at risk; stage B HF: pre-clinical, asymptomatic; stage C HF: past/present history of heart failure with symptoms; and stage D HF: end-stage heart failure.	

The recent report from the ISHLT, including patients from 1982 through 2014, showed that the median survival (time when 50% of the transplanted patients remain alive) was 20.6 years for infants, 17.3 years for children ages of 1 and 5 years, 14.6 years for children ages of 6 and 10 years, and 12.9 years for adolescents at the time of trans-plantation [37]. Heart transplant is still considered a potential option in pediatric patients with end stage heart failure to improve the quality of life and the overall survival.

CONSENT FOR PUBLICATION

Not applicable.

CONFLICT OF INTEREST

The authors confirm that this chapter contents have no conflict of interest.

ACKNOWLEDGEMENTS

Declared none.

REFERENCES

[1]   Abraham WT, Fisher WG, Smith AL, *et al.* Cardiac resynchronization in chronic heart failure. N Engl J Med 2002; 346(24): 1845-53.
      [http://dx.doi.org/10.1056/NEJMoa013168] [PMID: 12063368]

[2]   Young JB, Abraham WT, Smith AL, *et al.* Combined cardiac resynchronization and implantable cardioversion defibrillation in advanced chronic heart failure: the MIRACLE ICD Trial. JAMA 2003; 289(20): 2685-94.
      [http://dx.doi.org/10.1001/jama.289.20.2685] [PMID: 12771115]

[3]   Cleland JGF, Daubert J-C, Erdmann E, *et al.* The effect of cardiac resynchronization on morbidity and mortality in heart failure. N Engl J Med 2005; 352(15): 1539-49.
      [http://dx.doi.org/10.1056/NEJMoa050496] [PMID: 15753115]

[4]   van der Hulst AE, Delgado V, Blom NA, *et al.* Cardiac resynchronization therapy in paediatric and congenital heart disease patients. Eur Heart J 2011; 32(18): 2236-46.
      [http://dx.doi.org/10.1093/eurheartj/ehr093] [PMID: 21450719]

[5]   Dubin AM, Janousek J, Rhee E, *et al.* Resynchronization therapy in pediatric and congenital heart disease patients: an international multicenter study. J Am Coll Cardiol 2005; 46(12): 2277-83.
      [http://dx.doi.org/10.1016/j.jacc.2005.05.096] [PMID: 16360058]

[6]   Cecchin F, Frangini PA, Brown DW, *et al.* Cardiac resynchronization therapy (and multisite pacing) in pediatrics and congenital heart disease: five years experience in a single institution. J Cardiovasc Electrophysiol 2009; 20(1): 58-65.
      [http://dx.doi.org/10.1111/j.1540-8167.2008.01274.x] [PMID: 18775051]

[7]   Janousek J, Gebauer RA, Abdul-Khaliq H, *et al.* Cardiac resynchronisation therapy in paediatric and congenital heart disease: differential effects in various anatomical and functional substrates. Heart 2009; 95(14): 1165-71.
      [http://dx.doi.org/10.1136/hrt.2008.160465] [PMID: 19307198]

[8]   Strieper M, Karpawich P, Frias P, *et al.* Initial experience with cardiac resynchronization therapy for ventricular dysfunction in young patients with surgically operated congenital heart disease. Am J Cardiol 2004; 94(10): 1352-4.http://www.ncbi.nlm.nih.gov/pubmed/15541267 [Internet].
      [http://dx.doi.org/10.1016/j.amjcard.2004.07.134] [PMID: 15541267]

[9]   Janousek J, Tomek V, Chaloupecký VA, *et al.* Cardiac resynchronization therapy: a novel adjunct to the treatment and prevention of systemic right ventricular failure. J Am Coll Cardiol 2004; 44(9): 1927-31.
[http://dx.doi.org/10.1016/j.jacc.2004.08.044] [PMID: 15519030]

[10]   Cowburn PJ, Parker JD, Cameron DA, Harris L. Cardiac resynchronization therapy: retiming the failing right ventricle. J Cardiovasc Electrophysiol 2005; 16(4): 439-43.
[http://dx.doi.org/10.1046/j.1540-8167.2005.40590.x] [PMID: 15828891]

[11]   Jauvert G, Rousseau-Paziaud J, Villain E, *et al.* Effects of cardiac resynchronization therapy on echocardiographic indices, functional capacity, and clinical outcomes of patients with a systemic right ventricle. Europace 2009; 11(2): 184-90.
[http://dx.doi.org/10.1093/europace/eun319] [PMID: 19038975]

[12]   Zimmerman FJ, Starr JP, Koenig PR, Smith P, Hijazi ZM, Bacha EA. Acute hemodynamic benefit of multisite ventricular pacing after congenital heart surgery. Ann Thorac Surg 2003; 75(6): 1775-80.
[http://dx.doi.org/10.1016/S0003-4975(03)00175-9] [PMID: 12822614]

[13]   Bacha EA, Zimmerman FJ, Mor-Avi V, *et al.* Ventricular resynchronization by multisite pacing improves myocardial performance in the postoperative single-ventricle patient. Ann Thorac Surg 2004; 78(5): 1678-83.
[http://dx.doi.org/10.1016/j.athoracsur.2004.04.065] [PMID: 15511455]

[14]   Epstein AE, Dimarco JP, Ellenbogen KA, *et al.* ACC/AHA/HRS 2008 guidelines for Device-Based Therapy of Cardiac Rhythm Abnormalities: executive summary. Heart Rhythm 2008; 5(6): 934-55.
[http://dx.doi.org/10.1016/j.hrthm.2008.04.015] [PMID: 18534377]

[15]   Berul CI, Van Hare GF, Kertesz NJ, *et al.* Results of a multicenter retrospective implantable cardioverter-defibrillator registry of pediatric and congenital heart disease patients. J Am Coll Cardiol 2008; 51(17): 1685-91.
[http://dx.doi.org/10.1016/j.jacc.2008.01.033] [PMID: 18436121]

[16]   Silka MJ, Hardy BG, Menashe VD, Morris CD. A population-based prospective evaluation of risk of sudden cardiac death after operation for common congenital heart defects. J Am Coll Cardiol 1998; 32(1): 245-51.
[http://dx.doi.org/10.1016/S0735-1097(98)00187-9] [PMID: 9669277]

[17]   Rhee EK, Canter CE, Basile S, Webber SA, Naftel DC. Sudden death prior to pediatric heart transplantation: Would implantable defibrillators improve outcome? J Heart Lung Transplant 2007; 26(5)
[http://dx.doi.org/10.1016/j.healun.2007.02.005] [PMID: 17449412]

[18]   Mah D, Singh TP, Thiagarajan RR, *et al.* Incidence and risk factors for mortality in infants awaiting heart transplantation in the USA. J Heart Lung Transplant 2009; 28(12): 1292-8.
[http://dx.doi.org/10.1016/j.healun.2009.06.013] [PMID: 19782580]

[19]   Almond CSD, Thiagarajan RR, Piercey GE, *et al.* Waiting list mortality among children listed for heart transplantation in the United States. Circulation 2009; 119(5): 717-27.
[http://dx.doi.org/10.1161/CIRCULATIONAHA.108.815712] [PMID: 19171850]

[20]   Benden C, Edwards LB, Kucheryavaya AY, *et al.* The Registry of the International Society for Heart and Lung Transplantation: fifteenth pediatric lung and heart-lung transplantation report--2012. J Heart Lung Transplant 2012; 31(10): 1087-95.
[http://dx.doi.org/10.1016/j.healun.2012.08.005] [PMID: 22975098]

[21]   Adachi I, Fraser CD Jr. Mechanical circulatory support for infants and small children. Semin Thorac Cardiovasc Surg Pediatr Card Surg Annu 2011; 14(1): 38-44.
[http://dx.doi.org/10.1053/j.pcsu.2011.01.008] [PMID: 21444048]

[22]   Rossano JW, Shaddy RE. Heart failure in children: etiology and treatment. J Pediatr 2014; 165(2): 228-33.http://www.ncbi.nlm.nih.gov/pubmed/24928699 [Internet].
[http://dx.doi.org/10.1016/j.jpeds.2014.04.055] [PMID: 24928699]

[23]   Weinstein S, Bello R, Pizarro C, *et al.* The use of the Berlin Heart EXCOR in patients with functional single ventricle. J Thorac Cardiovasc Surg 2014; 147(2): 697-704.
[http://dx.doi.org/10.1016/j.jtcvs.2013.10.030] [PMID: 24290716]

[24]   Blume ED, Rosenthal DN, Rossano JW, *et al.* Outcomes of children implanted with ventricular assist devices in the United States: First analysis of the Pediatric Interagency Registry for Mechanical Circulatory Support (PediMACS). J Heart Lung Transplant 2016; 35(5): 578-84.
[http://dx.doi.org/10.1016/j.healun.2016.01.1227] [PMID: 27009673]

[25]   Adachi I. Continuous-flow ventricular assist device support in children: A paradigm change. J Thorac Cardiovasc Surg 2017; 154(4): 1358-61.
[http://dx.doi.org/10.1016/j.jtcvs.2017.02.082] [PMID: 28645826]

[26]   Nassar MS, Hasan A, Chila T, Schueler S, Pergolizzi C, Reinhardt Z, *et al.* Comparison of paracorporeal and continuous flow ventricular assist devices in children: Preliminary results Eur J Cardiothorac Surg 2017; 1;51(4): 709-14.
[http://dx.doi.org/10.1093/ejcts/ezx006]

[27]   Larose JA, Tamez D, Ashenuga M, Reyes C. Design concepts and principle of operation of the HeartWare ventricular assist system. ASAIO J 2010; 56(4): 285-9.
[http://dx.doi.org/10.1097/MAT.0b013e3181dfbab5] [PMID: 20559135]

[28]   Paridon SM, Mitchell PD, Colan SD, *et al.* A cross-sectional study of exercise performance during the first 2 decades of life after the Fontan operation. J Am Coll Cardiol 2008; 52(2): 99-107.
[http://dx.doi.org/10.1016/j.jacc.2008.02.081] [PMID: 18598887]

[29]   Paden ML, Rycus PT, Thiagarajan RR. Update and outcomes in extracorporeal life support. Semin Perinatol 2014; 38(2): 65-70.
[http://dx.doi.org/10.1053/j.semperi.2013.11.002] [PMID: 24580761]

[30]   Murphy DA, Hockings LE, Andrews RK, *et al.* Extracorporeal membrane oxygenation-hemostatic complications. Transfus Med Rev 2015; 29(2): 90-101.
[http://dx.doi.org/10.1016/j.tmrv.2014.12.001] [PMID: 25595476]

[31]   Esper SA. Extracorporeal Membrane Oxygenation. Adv Anesth 2017; 35(1): 119-43.
[http://dx.doi.org/10.1016/j.aan.2017.07.006] [PMID: 29103569]

[32]   Braun JP, Schroeder T, Buehner S, *et al.* Splanchnic oxygen transport, hepatic function and gastrointestinal barrier after normothermic cardiopulmonary bypass. Acta Anaesthesiol Scand 2004; 48(6): 697-703.
[http://dx.doi.org/10.1111/j.1399-6576.2004.00392.x] [PMID: 15196101]

[33]   Rossi M, Sganga G, Mazzone M, *et al.* Cardiopulmonary bypass in man: role of the intestine in a self-limiting inflammatory response with demonstrable bacterial translocation. Ann Thorac Surg 2004; 77(2): 612-8.
[http://dx.doi.org/10.1016/S0003-4975(03)01520-0] [PMID: 14759448]

[34]   Merrill ED, Schoeneberg L, Sandesara P, *et al.* Outcomes after prolonged extracorporeal membrane oxygenation support in children with cardiac disease--Extracorporeal Life Support Organization registry study. J Thorac Cardiovasc Surg 2014; 148(2): 582-8.
[http://dx.doi.org/10.1016/j.jtcvs.2013.09.038] [PMID: 24189317]

[35]   Kirk R, Dipchand AI, Edwards LB, Kucheryavaya AY, Benden C, Christie JD, *et al.* The Registry of the International Society for Heart and Lung Transplantation: Fifteenth Pediatric Heart Transplantation Report   2012 J Hear Lung Transplant [Internet] Elsevier Inc 2012; 31?(10): 1065-72.

[36]   Canter CE, Shaddy RE, Bernstein D, *et al.* Indications for heart transplantation in pediatric heart disease: a scientific statement from the American Heart Association Council on Cardiovascular Disease in the Young. Circulation 2007; 115(5): 658-76. [Internet].
[http://dx.doi.org/10.1161/CIRCULATIONAHA.106.180449] [PMID: 17261651]

[37]   Dipchand AI, Edwards LB, Kucheryavaya AY, *et al.* The registry of the International Society for Heart and Lung Transplantation: seventeenth official pediatric heart transplantation report--2014; focus theme: retransplantation. J Heart Lung Transplant 2014; 33(10): 985-95.
[http://dx.doi.org/10.1016/j.healun.2014.08.002] [PMID: 25242123]

SUBJECT INDEX

A

Abnormalities 2, 6, 8, 10, 12, 28, 36, 62, 64, 65, 69, 85, 97, 122, 162
  coronary 162
  electrophysiological 28
  microvascular 64
  morphological 69
  myocardial 12
  neuro-humoral 2
  papillary muscle 69
  rhythm 36
  valvular 85
ACE inhibitors 26, 30, 40, 44, 45, 46
  therapy 40
    prophylactic 40
Activation 2, 26, 45, 173
  fibrinolytic pathway 173
  neuro-hormonal 2
  neurohormonal system 26
  sympathetic 45
Adrenal 3
  cortex 3
  gland 3
Aerobic oxidation 42
Air embolism 166, 173
  inadvertent 166
Aldosterone antagonists (AA) 15, 45, 99
Amyloid fibrils 125
Amyloidosis 99, 124, 125
  cardiac 124, 125
Anaemia, severe 9
Anderson-fabry disease (AFD) 124
Angiontensin receptor blockers 99
Angiotensin-converting enzyme (ACE) 3, 40
Angiotensin-converting enzyme inhibitors (ACEIs) 14, 15, 16, 37, 38, 99
Angiotensin receptor blocker (ARB) 15, 40, 46, 99
Anthracyclines 27
Antihypertensive drugs 16
Antioxidant effect 46

Aortic stenosis 7, 27, 65
  severe 7, 27
Aortic valve 8, 9, 12, 15, 27, 43, 66, 67, 76, 101, 162
  disease 9, 12
  gradients 15
  obstruction 43
  pathology 101
Aortic valve stenosis 9, 14, 167
  critical 14
Apoptosis 4, 135
  cellular 135
Arrhythmias 10, 12, 13, 15, 17, 40, 42, 45, 46, 64, 66, 117, 120, 122, 134, 174
  life-threatening 134, 174
Arterial 2, 13, 161, 174
  baroreflexes 2
  blood gas 13
  blood gasses 161
  blood pressure 2
  oxygen desaturation, severe 174
Arteriolar vasoconstrictor 4
Aspirin 47
Atrial 4, 5, 8, 16, 34, 35, 36, 63, 66, 92, 129, 130
  arrhythmias 36, 92
  fibrillation 63, 66, 130
  fibrillation ablation 129
  fibrillation/flutter 66
  level communication 35
  natriuretic peptide (ANP) 4, 5
  septal communication 34
  septal defects (ASD) 8, 35
  tachyarrhythmias 16
Automated implantable cardiac defibrillator (AICD) 100, 115, 116

B

Balloon valvoplasty 14, 15
  aortic 15
Basal anteroseptal 122

Mohammad El Tahlawi (Ed.)
All rights reserved-© 2019 Bentham Science Publishers

www.ingramcontent.com/pod-product-compliance
Lightning Source LLC
Chambersburg PA
CBHW041659210326
41598CB00007B/467